Casualty Officer's
Handbook

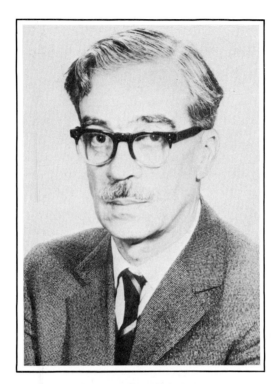

Maurice Ellis, F.R.C.S.
1904—1977

Casualty Officer's Handbook

FOURTH EDITION

DAVID H. WILSON
M.B., Ch.B.(Leeds), F.R.C.S.(Edin), D.T.M. & H.(Antwerp)
Senior Consultant, Accident and Emergency Department,
The General Infirmary at Leeds
Honorary Clinical Lecturer in Surgery, University of Leeds

MALCOLM H. HALL
M.R.C.S.(Eng), L.R.C.P.(London)
Consultant, Accident and Emergency Department,
Preston Royal Infirmary

BUTTERWORTHS
LONDON - BOSTON
Sydney - Wellington - Durban - Toronto

First published 1962
Second edition 1966
Third edition 1970
Reprinted 1971
Reprinted 1975
Reprinted 1977
Fourth edition 1979
Reprinted 1981

© Butterworth & Co (Publishers) Ltd 1979

British Library Cataloguing in Publication Data
Wilson, David H
    Casualty officer's handbook. — 4th ed.
    1. Wounds — Treatment   2. Medical emergencies
    I. Title   II. Hall, Malcolm H   III. Ellis,
    Maurice
    617'. 1   RD93   78–41189
    ISBN 0–407–00140–9

Typeset by Butterworth Litho Preparation Department
Printed and bound by Butler & Tanner Ltd, Frome, Somerset

Preface to the Fourth Edition

Before his death last year, Maurice Ellis asked us if we would prepare a new edition of his Casualty Officers' Handbook. We consider ourselves privileged to be his successors.

Since the third edition appeared, Accident and Emergency has become an established specialty within the National Health Service in the United Kingdom and a full career structure has been introduced. This development, which owes much to Maurice Ellis's pioneer work, is a reflection of his concern for the specialty and will remain a lasting tribute to his efforts.

In preparing this new edition we have kept to the same format but, because nine years have passed since the third edition was published, we have re-written much of the work and introduced new material in order to reflect the changing pattern of work within the Emergency Services. In keeping with the increasing importance of medical emergency care, we have included chapters on medical emergencies and paediatric problems, and we have extended the chapter on 'The Casualty Officer and the Law'. As in previous editions, we have sought to provide a handbook for junior doctors to help them deal with some of the many problems that they will face when they start to work in the Emergency Services. We hope that medical students and nurses will also find it helpful.

We wish to express our thanks to our secretaries, Miss Christine Whitehead and Mrs Barbara Parker, and to our colleagues who have made many helpful suggestions. We are also indebted to Mr Peter Hargreaves and the staff of the Medical Photographic Department of the General Infirmary at Leeds, and to Mr Peter Kilshaw and the staff of the Medical Illustration Department of Preston Royal Infirmary.

D. H. W. Leeds
M. H. H. Preston

Preface to the First Edition

This book has grown out of the teaching given to many students and junior Casualty Officers over the past ten years. Their questions and difficulties showed me that there seemed to be no book for them to consult for practical help in the management, diagnosis and treatment of the patient in front of them in the Casualty Department. Verbal instruction, therefore, became reinforced by written teaching on the more common injuries and emergencies seen in these patients. I was pleased, therefore, to accept the invitation from Butterworths to expand these written lectures into a practical handbook for Casualty Officers.

This handbook is designed to help the newly appointed Casualty Officer, or the House Surgeon and House Physician who have to do duty irregularly in the Casualty Department. Such recently qualified men and women are often left alone with no experienced senior available for advice on the management of patients in front of them. They need assistance in deciding what urgent help is required in the serious case, on how to manage the border-line case, and they require full details of the treatment of the less serious cases, which comprise the majority of patients treated. This book is not intended to replace standard textbooks on fractures, but does give details of the management of suspected fractures and the treatment required in the Casualty Department before the patient is passed on to the care of the fracture surgeon. Fractures, however, form no more than 15 per cent of the work of the Casualty Department. Some of the remaining patients need urgent life-saving procedures, but most require careful treatment of their wounds, sprains, abscesses and burns in the Casualty Department with equally careful follow-up treatment. This treatment and follow-up are described in detail.

Leeds, 1962   M. Ellis

Contents

1

Accidents

The Accident and Emergency Department exists for the reception and treatment of a wide variety of urgent medical and surgical conditions, and both public and hospital expect equally efficient and prompt treatment in severe and trivial cases alike. A survey of the 70 000 new patients coming each year to an A & E Department in an industrial city is valuable in giving an idea of the burden that has to be carried, the skills required for treatment and the equipment that should be available. The following figures show the age distribution and broad diagnostic categories:

Children	0–14 years	23%
Young people	15–24 years	24%
Adults	25–64 years	43%
Elderly	65+ years	10%

Accidents	71%
Acute medical conditions	15%
Acute surgical conditions	14%

Accident patients constitute by far the largest part of the work load. They can be divided into 4 categories:

1. Those requiring resuscitation — there is a danger to life and they may have multiple injuries probably requiring the services of several surgical specialities.
2. Those requiring in-patient treatment but with no immediate threat to life.
3. Those who can be treated as out-patients — even though their injuries may be moderately severe. For these patients the treatment will be carried out in full by the staff of the A & E Department.
4. Those with minor injuries — for whom efficient treatment is still required to prevent complications or unnecessarily long morbidity.

With each of these categories, a different kind of management is required. The type of patient in each category will therefore be described, together with the broad outlines of management. The treatment of burns in the A & E Department is described separately.

CATEGORY 1 – RESUSCITATION PATIENTS

Seriously injured patients with multiple injuries are few in relation to the less serious injuries which come to the A & E Department. The first time Accident Department doctors see such a patient they may find that their previous medical training has not prepared them to deal with this type of patient and they are often at a loss to know where to start in the management. Chapter 2 is therefore devoted to this important problem of the management of the severely injured patient.

CATEGORY 2 – REQUIRING IN-PATIENT TREATMENT

These patients will lie either in the province of the general surgeon or in one of the surgical specialities: orthopaedics, plastics, etc. Management in the A & E Department will consist of relieving pain, applying suitable splinting and temporary dressings, carrying out the necessary X-rays and establishing a provisional diagnosis. Head injury patients requiring admission to hospital, primarily for observation rather than immediate surgery, should be thoroughly examined to provide base-line information as described in Chapter 4; the management of patients in this category should be expeditious, but without the urgency of the first category.

CATEGORY 3 – TO BE TREATED AS OUT-PATIENTS

It is for patients in this category that the Accident Officer has the opportunity and is expected to show personal skill in the treatment of each individual patient. The reduction of dislocations, the manipulation of fractures and the suture of moderately severe wounds are all carried out in the A & E Department. In subsequent chapters, instructions for the treatment of these common injuries are given in detail with indications for the follow-up treatment.

In the management of these patients many pitfalls await the unwary. It would seem that most patients are only capable of complaining of one condition at a time, and they therefore direct the attention of the doctor to the most painful lesion, and often refuse to admit that any other part of the body has been injured. The discovery of one lesion

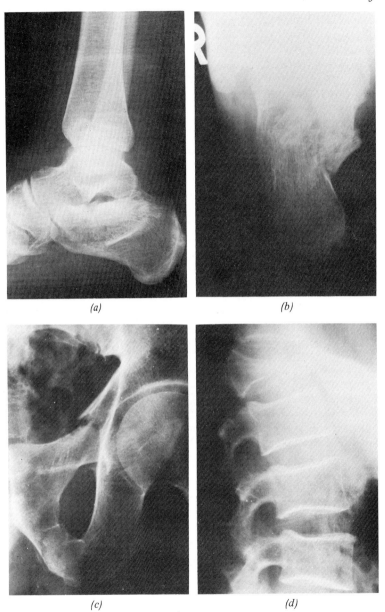

Figure 1.1.   X-Rays of a patient who fell 7 metres from a roof and landed on his heels. (a) and (b) Fractures of the os calcis. (c) Fracture of the hip. (d) Fracture of the lumbar spine

should not deter the doctor from excluding other conditions. For instance, a patient who has been knocked down by a motor car may only complain of an injury to the arm, and ignore the fact that the abdomen was hit at the same time causing trauma to the spleen or bowel. A fall from a height may have fractured the os calcis and at the same time have damaged the hip and the spine (*Figure 1.1*); the os calcis fracture is the most painful lesion and the other fractures may be missed. These accidents may not be so immediately dangerous to life as those in category 1 but, unless there is an adequate physical examination, treatment may be arranged on an out-patient basis for the most painful lesion when the other more serious lesions require admission to hospital.

CATEGORY 4 – MINOR INJURIES

The number of patients in category 4 will probably exceed the combined total of all 3 previous categories. The minor nature of the conditions should not be made an excuse for an inadequate examination or treatment. Many of the patients are wage-earners and wish to be away from work for the minimum period. If adequate supervision and skill are not exercised, complications, such as sepsis and the breaking down of wounds, may prolong absence from work by several weeks. If each patient is away from work one week less, the saving to industry and to the economy of the country will be immense. The saving to the hospital by the reduced bill for the dressings will also be considerable. To achieve such a result it is imperative that every patient be seen by a doctor. If the treatment is delegated, the doctor must be satisfied that the person to whom he delegates it is adequately trained and competent to carry out the instructions and has fully understood the doctor's intentions. A treatment routine must be established with the co-operation of the nursing staff, the correct instructions must be available and the entire staff of the department must take a pride in the quality of their work.

IT IS ALSO IMPERATIVE THAT AN ADEQUATE RECORD IS MADE AND KEPT OF EVERY PATIENT, HOWEVER TRIVIAL THEIR COMPLAINT MAY APPEAR TO BE; SUCH NOTES MUST BE CONCISE BUT ACCURATE. THEY WILL NOT ONLY HAVE CLINICAL SIGNIFICANCE BUT THEY MAY ALSO ASSUME MEDICO-LEGAL IMPORTANCE AT A LATER DATE.

2

The Management of the Severely Injured Patient

AT THE SCENE OF THE ACCIDENT

Ideally, the management of severely injured patients should start at the scene of the accident and ambulance crews are now trained for this task. The most important single item of management is the care of the patient's respiration. In the unconscious patient the airway may be blocked by the tongue falling backwards, or by secretions, blood, vomit, false teeth or other foreign bodies. Having removed all extraneous material from the mouth, the jaw is pulled forwards and held until the patient can be turned into the semi-prone or 'recovery position'.

1. The airway

In the recovery position secretions will drain to the outside and the jaw will fall forward (*Figure 2.1*). Even in the conscious patient the airway may be partially obstructed and the patient unable to clear it by coughing; ambulances now carry suction apparatus and pharyngeal airways to deal with this problem. The value of training ambulance men to pass an endo-tracheal tube at the scene of the accident is still under discussion.

2. Open wounds

After taking care of the respiration, temporary sterile dressings should be applied to open wounds. The use of a tourniquet to control arterial bleeding is not encouraged: a local pressure pad and bandage is re-commended. The pulse should be checked and an estimate made of the volume of blood lost at the scene of the accident. Inflatable splints are not only valuable for supporting fractures in the distal half of the limbs but also because they will stop bleeding; they should be blown up by mouth and released temporarily every hour if the journey is prolonged.

5

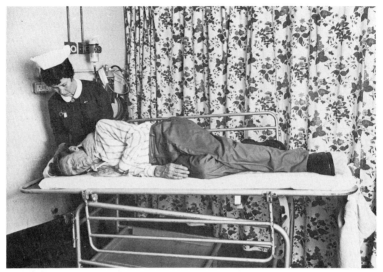

Figure 2.1.   The recovery position. The patient must not be left unattended

3. Analgesia and splints

In order to ease the pain when applying splints and moving the patient at the scene of the accident, analgesia can be given by an entonox apparatus which delivers 50 per cent oxygen and 50 per cent nitrous oxide. The apparatus is difficult to use if there are severe facial injuries and should never be used in the presence of fire or sparks from metal cutting equipment because of the risk of an explosion. Fractured upper limbs can be supported by lightly bandaging them to the chest wall. If one leg is fractured the other will serve as a splint, but if both legs are injured external supports must be applied. If the patient is trapped and a spinal injury is suspected, a spinal board should be used to support the back and neck while extricating the patient.

4. Moving the patient

Considerable skill is necessary for handling and moving patients. A stout canvas carrying sheet can be unrolled under the patient's body and poles introduced into the side folds for lifting. These sheets should be interchangeable between hospitals and the ambulance service so that the

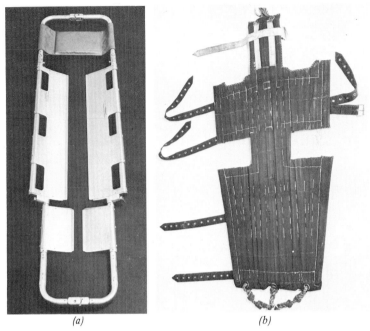

(a)   *(b)*

Figure 2.2. (a) Scoop stretcher. (b) Neil Robertson stretcher

patient can remain on the same carrying sheet until he reaches the ward, the ambulance being re-equipped with another carrying sheet from the hospital supply. For patients with displaced fractures, a metal scoop stretcher may be preferable to give support to the injured limbs and occasionally, in difficult circumstances, a Neil Robertson stretcher is indicated (*Figure 2.2*).

5. Transport to hospital

If there are any witnesses to the accident, enquiries should be made before leaving the scene to find out if the patient has been unconscious, and to obtain a brief account of the accident.

After moving the patient into the ambulance, the airway and pulse must be checked again. If the pulse is weak or the patient cyanosed, oxygen should be administered during the journey to hospital. Assuming the ambulance is equipped with a radio-telephone, the receiving hospital should be warned that the patient (or patients) is on the way, if possible giving an estimated time of arrival. Transport, by road or by air, should be as rapid as possible without causing any further trauma to the patient. Throughout the journey, observations must be made on the respiration, pulse and level of consciousness. If the expertise is available, an intravenous infusion can be started.

RECEPTION OF THE PATIENT AT HOSPITAL

In the reception bay

When the A & E Department of the hospital receives notification of the expected arrival of the injured patient, a reception team should be made available — doctors, nurses and porters. The equipment the team require is as follows:

1. A resuscitation trolley of which the surface can be raised or lowered at either end, is radio-translucent and has a device for holding X-ray cassettes under the surface. The trolley should also have a holder for an oxygen cylinder, a drip attachment and a wire basket for the patient's clothes and property.
2. An oxygen cylinder with mask and flowmeter.
3. A bag containing a suitable selection of airway tubes, a laryngoscope, cuffed endotracheal tubes and other equipment for endotracheal intubation.
4. A portable suction apparatus (*Figure 2.3*).
5. A spare carrying sheet and poles.

On arrival of the ambulance, the doctor should immediately check the patient's respiration. In the unconscious patient, if the airway is obstructed, endotracheal intubation and tracheal toilet may be performed in the ambulance and positive pressure respiration started if necessary; but there should be no undue delay before the patient is wheeled to the resuscitation room.

IN THE RESUSCITATION ROOM

A modern resuscitation room must be warm, well-lit, private, have adequate floor space, be fully equipped with the necessary apparatus including X-ray, have piped gases and suction, and be in telephone

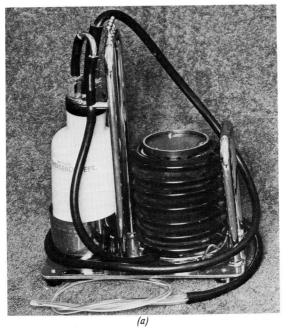

(a)

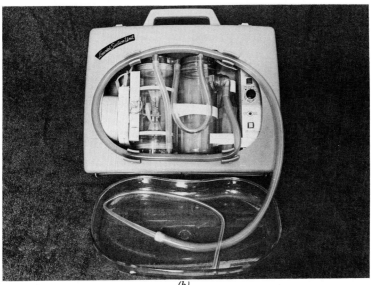

(b)

Figure 2.3. (a) Foot-operated suction apparatus. (b) Battery-operated portable suction unit

communication with the rest of the A & E Department and the hospital (*Figure 2.4*). The quick and efficient resuscitation of seriously injured patients requires team work. Delegation of duties among the members

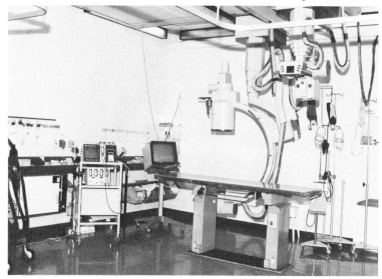

Figure 2.4.   Resuscitation room with facilities for intubation, ventilation, fluid replacement, monitoring and radiology

of the team should be done by the senior doctor. The various aspects of the work are listed below and in order of priority but ideally they should run concurrently.

1. Care of the airway

If the lungs do not receive an adequate supply of oxygen all other aspects of resuscitation are useless. Respiratory obstruction can occur in conscious or unconscious patients. In the majority of cases, positioning the patient and, if necessary, sucking out the mouth and pharynx is sufficient. In the unconscious patient the use of a pharyngeal airway may be indicated. If there is blood in the air passages it may clot in the airway and intubation with a cuffed tube will be necessary. Quick and effective endotracheal intubation demands a certain amount of skill and the head of the department must ensure that all the medical staff are trained in this procedure. If cyanosis is not relieved by intubation and oxygen therapy, the possibility of an intrathoracic injury must be considered. If oxygenation of the blood is impaired a sample of arterial blood in a heparinized syringe must be taken for blood gas analysis.

2a. Prevention or treatment of shock by fluid replacement

To make an initial assessment of the need for fluid replacement it may be necessary to cut the clothing along the seams to avoid the trauma of undressing the patient. As this is done, base-line information is recorded of pulse, blood pressure, respiration, temperature and level of consciousness; this will be a guide as to whether fluid replacement is indicated. The ambulance attendant's report is also helpful at this point. Were the circumstances of the accident such that internal bleeding is likely? How much blood was lost at the scene of the accident and during the ambulance journey? How much blood has been soaked up by the patient's clothing and the First Aid dressings? The volume of internal bleeding into the limbs is related to the swelling. A fracture of the shaft of the femur will result in approximately one litre of blood being extruded into the soft tissues of the thigh. A major disruption of the pelvis with palpable instability may cause 2–3 litres of blood to be lost to the circulation. Similarly, the thoracic and abdominal cavities can each accommodate 3 or more litres of blood. The presence of such massive internal haemorrhage should always be considered when the patient fails to respond to an apparently adequate volume of fluid replacement.

If the extent of the injuries is such that circulatory collapse is likely to develop then fluid replacement must be begun immediately. It is much easier to introduce an intravenous canula when the peripheral veins are well filled; once they have collapsed, even with a satisfactorily placed canula, it may be difficult to obtain an adequate rate of transfusion and cannulation of the subclavian vein may become necessary.

There is no one sign, nor any single clinical measurement, on which to make a diagnosis of shock. It is a composite picture of a cold, anxious, pale, sweating patient with rapid shallow respiration, the pulse rate is raised and the pulse volume reduced, the blood pressure is low and the peripheral veins are collapsed. This situation demands immediate transfusion of warmed blood under pressure, possibly at multiple sites. A central venous pressure monitor will be useful in gauging the rate and volume of transfusion.

For patients in either category, those in whom shock is anticipated and those in whom it is already present, a sample of blood should be taken for grouping and cross-matching as soon as the intravenous canula is introduced. The quantity of blood to be requested will depend on the clinical assessment.

The first choice for the transfusion site is a forearm vein, but injuries or other circumstances may make it necessary to use the external jugular vein or a scalp vein in a baby. When the peripheral veins are all collapsed either a 'cut-down' into the long saphenous vein at the ankle or in the femoral triangle is indicated, or subclavian cannulation.

2b. Choice of fluid

There is considerable difference of opinion as to the type of fluid to use. The choice lies between electrolyte solutions, plasma substitues, plasma and whole blood.

Electrolyte solutions: normal saline of Hartman's solution is usually employed to establish the drip and in less severe cases may be all that is necessary. They can also be used for fluid replacement until fully grouped and cross-matched blood is available provided the blood pressure remains at a satisfactory level.

Plasma substitutes can perform 2 functions: those containing molecules of a relatively small size (about 30 000 molecular weight) are valuable for the restoration of the peripheral circulation in tissue of doubtful viability; those with larger molecules (60 000–70 000 molecular weight) are used to maintain or restore the circulating blood volume. The dextrans have been used for these purposes for many years but they have the disadvantage of causing difficulties in blood cross-matching if given before taking the blood sample from the patient. The recent introduction of a solution using a modified gelatin molecule of relatively low molecular weight appears to have overcome this problem.

Plasma: reconstituted plasma may carry the risk of transmitting serum hepatitis and plasma protein fraction is to be preferred. It is expensive to produce and its use should be restricted to cases where there is a biological indication, as in the treatment of burns.

Whole blood is preferable to other replacement fluids when the combined external and internal blood loss in a formerly healthy patient is estimated to be greater than 20 per cent of the circulating blood volume (*Figure 2.5*). Group O Rhesus negative blood is in short supply and should only be used when time does not permit cross-matching procedures to be carried out. In a severe emergency group O Rhesus positive blood can be used for male patients (or post-menopausal women) for whom this factor is less significant.

Full compatibility tests can take as long as 2 hours and a decision may have to be taken to use blood which has been grouped but not cross-matched. When blood is being transfused a doctor must check each unit before it is administered.

In the A & E Department it is not unknown for two patients bearing the same name to be injured in the same accident, and both require blood transfusion. Identification must therefore include both the patient's name and the hospital registration number. The reaction of the patient to the transfusion must be recorded at regular intervals and failure to respond will suggest continued internal bleeding.

13

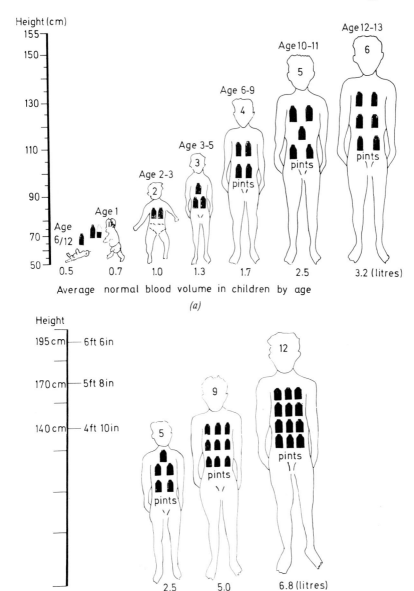

Figure 2.5. (a) Average normal blood volume in children by age and height
(b) Average normal blood volume in adults by height

3. Physical examination of the whole body

The respiration and circulation are now under control and a more detailed examination of the patient can be undertaken. The history of the accident is important. The ambulance man's account should allow an assessment to be made of the violence and the various forces to which the patient was exposed. Following a high velocity road accident, it is always wise to assume that the patient will have sustained a deceleration type of injury such as a rupture of the aorta, even if the initial examination is apparently normal. Imprints on the skin of a seat belt, clothing or a steering wheel must be noted and strongly suggest the likelihood of damage to internal viscera. From a clinical point of view the abbreviation 'RTA' for a road traffic accident is meaningless without further details. Patients injured in explosions will probably have sustained damage to the ear drums and lungs, and this again will be suggested by the history of the accident.

Because the conscious patient does not necessarily give a comprehensive account of his symptoms he requires a full examination. The unconscious patient, being unable to guide the doctor, must be similarly examined. It is advisable in the conscious patient and essential in the unconscious patient, to repeat the physical examination at regular intervals until the extent and progress of the injuries allows the correct decision to be made for their management. All the physical findings must be recorded and the time noted. A member of the resuscitation team can act as a scribe writing down not only the history and the details of the physical examination, but also a record of blood samples despatched and transfusions and injections given to the patient.

The physical examination should follow an established routine. Injuries to the head and trunk carry the greatest threat to life in the first few hours, and so are accorded priority. The presence of a spinal injury cannot be excluded at this stage and all handling of the patient must be done carefully with this possibility in mind. Details of the examination and treatment of the head, trunk and limbs are described in the appropriate chapters. The possibility of the patient having a pre-existing illness or an acute medical disorder before the accident must not be overlooked. It is also helpful to know if the patient was receiving medication or taking illicit drugs, as this may affect the physical signs or alter the reaction to the trauma or its treatment. The nature and extent of injuries to the limbs will have been noted, and when dressings and splints are applied the fingers and toes must be left exposed to allow a continuous assessment of the circulation in all 4 limbs. Blankets and sheets should not be allowed to hide these areas.

Ideally, X-ray examination should be done in the resuscitation room. In the unsatisfactory event of this not being possible, then the process of resuscitation and the necessary regular physical observations must continue in the X-Ray Department. Recent experience with fluoroscopy and image intensification in the resuscitation room has proved to be of immense value. The integrity of the cervical spine can be demonstrated. A dynamic picture of cardio—respiratory action is obtained. Fractures, dislocations and foreign bodies are quickly located and the whole comprehensive survey takes only 1—2 minutes.

4. The use of drugs

A patient may have sustained a major injury but will not necessarily complain of pain. The only indication for the use of analgesia is a complaint of pain. Entonox will give temporary analgesia during the application of splints and well-applied spints are, of themselves, immediately effective in reducing pain. It is preferable not to use other analgesics because they may mask the patient's symptoms and possibly depress respiration. Pupillary signs will be less reliable and the level of consciousness may be modified. If further analgesia is necessary, drugs must be administered intravenously in small doses which can be repeated when indicated. Either morphine (5—10 mg) or pethidine (50—100 mg) in an adult are effective but each carry their particular disadvantages. The newer synthetic analgesics have still to establish themselves in emergency care; similarly, the use of corticosteroids in the treatment of shock is still under evaluation. Patients on long-term medication such as insulin, steroids, beta-blockers, digitalis, etc., will require special consideration during their resuscitation and expert assistance may be required for their management. The use of antibiotics and tetanus prophylaxis in the treatment of wounds is discussed in Chapter 18.

5. Arrangements for definitive treatment

Several specialist units may be involved in the management of any one patient. Priorities in treatment will be decided by these specialists, but it remains the responsibility of the accident and emergency doctor to ensure that the overall well-being of the patient is not jeopardized by excessive concentration on any one injury. The departmental routine must ensure that each patient has his own unique registration details and these should be attached to the patient by a wrist band. This registration number must be used on all forms and biological samples, and the departmental staff must make sure that the results of all laboratory investigations are transmitted to the specialists involved in the patient's definitive treatment. When the patient is transported to the ward or operating theatre, he should be accompanied by a doctor or a nurse and it may be wise to have a portable suction apparatus available during the journey.

6. Interviews with relatives

Every A & E Department should have a quiet, pleasantly furnished room where patients' relatives can wait and eventually be told the nature of the injuries, or occasionally of the fatal outcome of the accident. The room should have a handbasin, mirror and telephone. It is important for medical and nursing staff to make sure of the identity of the people in the interview room and their relationship with the patient, before passing on personal details or catastrophic news. Similarly, information received from relatives immediately following an accident may not necessarily be accurate and, if possible, confirmation should be discretely obtained before acting upon it. The onerous task of informing relatives of the fatal outcome of an accident must be done with compassion and sympathy and is a task for the senior doctor and nurse on duty.

3

X-Rays in the Emergency Department

An Accident and Emergency Department cannot function without a 24 hour, 7 days a week X-ray service. Ideally, X-ray facilities should be available within the Accident Department but, at the very least, it should have easy and rapid access to the hospital's main X-Ray Unit.

The Accident Officer has the responsibility of deciding which patients should be referred for X-ray examination and he must be able to interpret films produced by the radiographer. Senior staff may not always be available to assist in the interpretation of X-rays and the Casualty Officer must train himself into a standard routine to avoid missing less obvious fractures or abnormalities that may show on a film. He must realize that X-rays are merely shadows and that they are not of themselves any more important than any other investigation. Many fractures are missed because the Accident Officer fails to relate the clinical picture presented by the patient to the shadows on the X-ray film. Before referring a patient for X-ray examination, he should have reached some tentative conclusion, based on the history and the examination, about the possibility or otherwise of the X-ray showing an abnormality. The importance of making a clinical diagnosis and using the X-ray film to support his conclusions cannot be over-emphasized. He should also realize that the taking of an X-ray picture does subject the patient to a small dose of ionizing radiation, that it is expensive and that it may fail to show abnormalities. The indications for X-ray examination must be based on clinical grounds alone and other aspects of a patient's condition should not, in general, influence his decision to order such an examination. Provided careful consideration has been given to the medical management of the patient and that his findings and conclusions are fully documented on the record card, a good defence can be made against a subsequent claim for negligence. If, however, a fracture is missed because of a failure to take an X-ray, when the history, examination and conclusions are inadequately recorded, it is very difficult to provide any meaningful defence against a charge of negligence.

17

A well organized Accident Department should have a system in operation designed to pick up fractures which the junior doctors may miss. A simple and effective system involves the scrutiny of the X-ray reports received back from the Consultant Radiologist in conjunction with the patient's record card. In this way steps can be taken to call back to the hospital for further examination patients who are reported as having sustained a fracture, but in whom the junior doctor failed to recognize the abnormality. In some patients all that may be necessary is to advise the General Practitioner about the abnormality; this is essential when the patient lives a considerable distance away from the hospital.

EXAMINATION OF X-RAY FILMS

1. An efficient viewing screen is essential. Ideally, this should have a high intensity bulb built in and controlled by a switch, against which denser areas can be scrutinized. A highly efficient method of missing minor abnormalities is to make a casual examination by holding the film up to a window or to one of the lights in the department.
2. The doctor should satisfy himself that the film does belong to the patient under consideration and that the correct side of the body has been X-rayed. The film should always be placed against the viewing screen in its proper anatomical orientation.
3. The darker area around the outline of the bones should be inspected, if necessary against the high intensity spot, to exclude the presence of foreign bodies or surgical emphysema. The overall texture of the bones should be considered and abnormalities noted.
4. The cortex of the bones should then be followed round, if necessary using a finger or point of a pen to trace the outline. A minimum of 2 views, taken at appropriate angles, is essential in order to diagnose a fracture. The film should never be marked in any way; the presence of an arrow or other indication of abnormality on a film draws the eye of the observer to that area and can result in other injuries being overlooked.
5. In most cases the fracture or other abnormality can be recognized with ease, but in certain injuries no abnormality may be seen. If the clinical presentation indicates that a fracture should be present, then the patient should be treated for the injury and re-X-rayed in 10 to 14 days. By this time the fracture line will be clearly visible or, in children, callus will be present (*Figure 3.1*).

Certain areas of the body present major difficulties to the inexperienced doctor and it is only through careful self-training and the rigid adherence

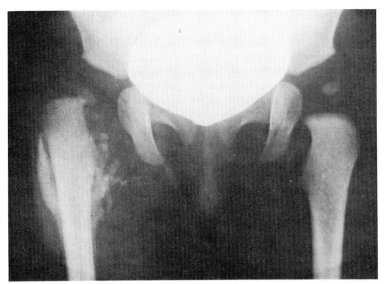

Figure 3.1.   Hypertrophic callus around injury to upper end of femur in a young baby.   No fracture can be seen but the large mass of callus indicates that bony damage has occurred.   In view of the altered relationship between the epiphysis and the metaphysis of the neck of the femur, the injury probably involved the neck of the femur

to a routine that proficiency may be developed. The areas which give rise to particular difficulties in interpretation are:

Fractures of the spine.
Fractures of the os calcis.
Fractures of the scaphoid.
Dislocations of the semilunar.
Fractures of the maxillo-facial skeleton.

These are discussed in the appropriate chapters.

Apart from missing a fracture, the film may be wrongly interpreted, for example a Smith's fracture may be labelled as a Colles' fracture because of failure to establish the anterior or posterior surfaces of the bone.

In children the bone may be tender but no fracture may be visible. A later X-ray, however, frequently confirms the original clinical assessment.

Congenital abnormalities, for example a bipartite patella, are a frequent cause of over-treatment; the junior doctor should make himself aware of the common developmental abnormalities that he is likely to see.

Referred pain can also result in fractures being missed. Pain in the knee joint when the pathology is in the hip area is a common example of this situation. Others include the referral of pain from spinal injuries to the abdomen (this may simulate intra-abdominal lesions) and bilateral shoulder or arm pain from injuries of the cervical spine.

The interpretation of chest X-rays is difficult. Each bony structure should be considered individually. The ribs should be traced, using a finger as a guide, and careful attention must be given to those areas where tenderness is present. The position of the heart and trachea must be

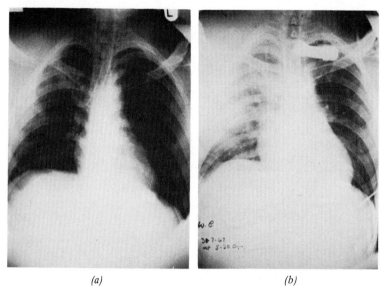

(a)   *(b)*

Figure 3.2.   Chest X-rays taken (a) shortly after, and (b) 6 hours after a chest injury. The initial film shows only slight mottling of the right lung; 6 hours later extensive mottling, due to pulmonary contusion, is clearly visible

assessed and the apices should be studied for evidence of pneumothorax. Opacity at the base may indicate a haemothorax and slight alterations in the texture of the lungs may indicate a pulmonary contusion. X-Ray examination an hour or two later will show pronounced mottling, indicative of haemorrhage in the pulmonary tissues (*Figure 3.2*).

In the seriously injured patient, there is little point in X-raying obvious limb fractures. Clinical assessment will enable an estimate of blood loss to be made, and detailed radiographic studies for the purpose of treatment can be left until the patient's condition has improved. If the patient's condition is serious, particularly if the limb injuries do not appear to provide an adequate explanation for his condition, the possibility of a concealed blood loss must be considered and X-ray examination of the pelvic girdle using, if necessary, a portable machine, should be carried out. Patients with major fractures of the pelvic girdle may require very large transfusions and X-ray examination is necessary in order that an estimate of the blood loss may be made. X-Ray examination of the chest may reveal a haemothorax or a haemopneumothorax. Intrathoracic blood loss can be assessed and other evidence may be found to account for the patient's altered respiratory state. Films taken under emergency conditions may not be technically perfect and, when the patient's condition has improved, these areas should be re-X-rayed (*see Figures 7.8* and *7.9*).

A fracture can be missed at the initial examination in patients with multiple injuries. The patient's complaints tend to be localized to the more significant injuries and minor fractures may be overlooked; repeated thorough clinical and radiographic examination is required to avoid this hazard. The unconscious patient, being unable to complain, is a particular clinical risk from this point of view and patients injured in high velocity impacts require comprehensive X-ray examination, which should include the cervical spine, thorax and frequently the pelvis.

4

Head Injuries

Patients with head injuries form an appreciable amount of the work of any Accident and Emergency Department. In general, the management of these patients is straightforward but there are some patients in whom the assessment presents difficulties, largely because of the risk of intracranial haemorrhage developing some hours after they have been seen in the department. These patients, who may appear to be normal when they are seen, will die if treatment is delayed, whereas surgery, if carried out immediately the signs and symptoms appear, offers the prospect of complete recovery. The initial responsibility of managing patients with so-called minor head injuries remains with the Accident Officer. It is a responsibility which cannot be passed on to more senior people and it is only by following a regular routine that catastrophies can be avoided. Whatever system is adopted, it is inevitable that errors of judgement will be made from time to time, but a systematized approach will do much to avoid missing the relatively uncommon intracranial bleed.

The junior doctor should realize that, in the context of the Emergency Department, head injuries cannot be subdivided into easily classifiable groups: they present as different degrees of the same injury, and a patient with an apparently minor head injury can very rapidly change into a patient who may die without immediate surgery. From a practical point of view there are only 2 groups of head injury patients: those in whom there is no history of unconsciousness and those in whom there is a history of unconsciousness. The duration of the loss of consciousness is irrelevant in terms of management. The presence or absence of fractures in the skull, while important, is of less significance than evidence of damage to the patient's brain. In the majority of head injuries, treatment is based upon this latter factor; extensive linear fractures, however spectacular, do not require treatment. Compound fractures require the normal surgical procedures for this type of injury, but the ultimate well-being of the patient depends on the presence or absence of cerebral damage, and diagnosis and treatment, in the absence of compound fractures, is primarily the management of the cerebral state of the patient.

In no group of injuries is the history of such great significance as in these patients. One of the major advances in recent years in A & E Units has been the training of ambulance personnel to give the staff an accurate history of the time and circumstances of the accident, and the patient's condition between the accident and his arrival at hospital. These details should be obtained about any patient who presents at a department, even though the injury appears trivial. The time and history of the occurrence can usually be obtained from parents, if the patient is a child, or other witnesses. Information about changes in the patient's level of consciousness at the time of, and immediately after, the accident, and during the journey to hospital should be obtained. This must be recorded on the case sheet because it may form the basis on which a subsequent decision to operate on the patient is taken.

Assessing loss of consciousness can present difficulties. Many patients, after a blow on the head, are dazed for short periods and, when asked, they say that they have been unconscious for a short period. When witnesses to the occurrence are asked they indicate that the patient was not unconscious. Similarly, untrained observers frequently state that a patient has been unconscious, yet on questioning further it is clear that this was not the case and that the patient was either unsteady or only confused by the accident. In order to avoid inaccurate assessments based on misinformation supplied by unskilled observers, it is wise to obtain a factual account about the patient's condition and reactions after the accident. This can be recorded in the notes and will mean the same thing to later observers.

If there are no witnesses to the accident and the patient states he has been unconscious, it is best to take the patient through his actions and memories for the period immediately before and after the accident. In this way a gap in their memory, composed of retrograde and post-traumatic amnesia, can be established. If this period is more than one or two minutes, loss of consciousness can be assumed and disposal of the patient is based on this feature.

LEVEL OF CONSCIOUSNESS

Consciousness implies an awareness and an ability to react in an appropriate manner to one's surroundings. From the time of the doctor's first contact with a patient who has sustained a head injury, he should be seeking to exclude changes in the patient's state of consciousness. Confusion, disorientation, irritability, inappropriate responses and reactions to various stimuli, repetitive questioning of staff, restlessness and, on occasions, violence towards the staff, all indicate that there has been cerebral damage and that admission will be necessary. A record should be made of the patient's reactions and responses to the various situations at the time of the initial assessment and at intervals when the assessment is repeated.

In other patients there is a varying degree of absence of purposeful response to stimulation and it is the doctor's duty to assess the level of consciousness. This is done by applying stimuli of a varying degree of intensity and noting the patient's response. Minor stimuli consist of shouting instructions in the patient's ear, moving or lifting a limb or shining a light in the eye. If these fail to produce a response, gentle pinching of the skin of the forearm, pressure on the supra-orbital nerve or squeezing the tendon achilles can be tried. The patient's response to painful procedures such as the application of splints to fractured limbs, injection or setting up intravenous drips, should be noted.

An unresponsive patient is one who fails to respond to any degree of stimulation. This indicates a major head injury and close observation and repeated examinations to assess progress will be necessary.

It will be observed that no attempt has been made to group patients into conscious and unconscious sections. This is because such an artificial classification is of little help in the management of the individual patient. A patient who appears to be 'conscious' may, on questioning, make a totally irrelevant reply; whereas a patient who appears to be 'unconscious' may take a highly appropriate movement, such as pushing the hand away when his arm is pinched. Both these patients could be labelled conscious or unconscious depending on the individual observer and the use of these terms in the initial documentation is inadvisable.

The on-going management of a head injury depends on regular assessment of the level of consciousness. The patient who initially responds only to painful stimuli and later responds to shouting is showing an improvement, whereas the patient who responds to questions in a normal voice and subsequently fails to respond except to maximal stimulation, is obviously deteriorating. The speed at which improvement or deterioration takes place is also of importance, especially when a well orientated patient rapidly becomes less responsive. This strongly suggests a progressive lesion which, in the context of head injuries, is probably an intracranial haemorrhage.

EXAMINATION

The head is inspected for bruises, wounds or other evidence of injury. Palpation of the scalp is helpful in the identification of blunt trauma to the vault.

In the absence of a laceration which has allowed blood to trickle down externally, bleeding from the nose or ears usually indicates fractures of the base of the skull in the frontal or temporal regions. Leakage of cerebrospinal fluid from the nose is not easily seen in the Emergency Department due to admixture with blood; it is usually recognized a day or two later in the wards when the bleeding has stopped.

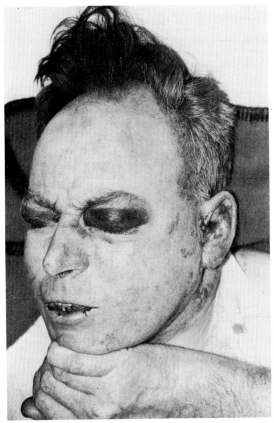

Figure 4.1.   Typical appearance of patient with fractured base of skull, showing black eyes and bleeding from left ear and mouth

Bruising, starting in the upper eyelids and spreading downwards, associated with subconjunctival haemorrhage extending backwards into the orbit, is indicative of a fracture of the base of the skull (*Figure 4.1*).

The state of the pupils is of great importance. Immediately following the injury there may be some degree of inequality. This is, however, only of short duration and, by the time the patient arrives in the department, stabilization will have occurred. The size and reaction of each pupil to light should be noted; if the patient will co-operate, eye movements should be tested. Occasionally paralysis of the extra-ocular muscles will be found and nystagmus, either horizontal or vertical, will be present.

If practical, other cranial nerves should be tested.

The presence of convulsions or other involuntary muscle movements should be noted. In the conscious patient the limbs should be examined for evidence of paralysis. In the unconscious patient an estimate of the tone of the limbs should be made. This can be measured by assessing the resistance of the limbs to passive movements, or alternatively by lifting the limb and allowing it to drop back on to the trolley.

The limb reflexes and the plantar responses should also be tested.

Neck rigidity or restriction of straight leg raising suggests meningeal irritation and is frequently found in fractures of the posterior fossa.

Other injuries

The patient should be examined for the presence of other injuries and diseases, some of which may confuse the diagnosis and others which may modify the patient's response to the head injury. The possibility of a cervical spine injury should not be overlooked after road traffic accidents.

ASSESSMENT

Initial assessment of the patient is possible at this stage. It is made by balancing the disturbances in the level of consciousness against the clinical findings. The larger the disturbance of consciousness and the more marked the neurological abnormalities, the greater the degree of injury to the brain and associated structures. Subsequent management and disposal of the patient depends on this assessment and the prognosis is also related to these initial findings. Many permutations of the history and examination are possible, but several well defined groups, with differing management, can be recognized:

1. The patient with dazing following the injury, who has recovered by the time of the examination without exhibiting any neurological abnormalities or loss of memory for the incident, can be allowed home after an hour or two of observation in the department.
2. The patient who has suffered a loss of consciousness should be admitted to hospital for observation. If there is still a disturbance of consciousness by the time the patient reaches hospital,

considerable cerebral damage may have occurred but, apart from routine attention to the airway, no specific treatment is required in the Emergency Department.

Of greater significance is the patient who has been unconscious after the accident but who is essentially normal on arrival. If there are no abnormalities, particularly of the pupils, it is unusual for further problems to arise but, from time to time, some patients in this group, after an initial normal examination, begin to show a deterioration in their level of consciousness. If this is associated with gradual dilatation and ultimate fixation of a pupil, followed by similar progressive changes in the contralateral pupil, the patient is suffering from an acute extradural haemorrhage. Recovery depends on evacuating the haematoma before the contra-lateral pupil becomes fixed and dilated. Once the contra-lateral pupil starts to dilate, decompression must be carried out within 15 to 20 minutes in an adult patient to prevent irreversible changes developing. Up to the age of 25 years, there can still be good recovery following a short period with bilateral dilated pupils. This improved prognosis adds even greater urgency to the surgery, which is such that, if it is not possible to operate upon the patient immediately in the main theatre, the decompression must be carried out in the emergency theatre.

The haemorrhage may be from either a meningeal artery or vein. It is of little matter from which vessel the haemorrhage occurs; the primary requisite is to allow the haematoma to drain through a hole in the skull. Once this has been done, the haematoma is decompressed, urgency is removed and the patient can then be transferred to the main theatre for enlargement of the burr hole to arrest the haemorrhage.

3. The patient who exhibits fixed dilatation of one or both pupils from the time of the accident, associated with a marked impairment of consciousness, has sustained major cerebral damage. Such a patient may or may nor recover, but surgery is not indicated, except in a child or young adult.

In summary, unconsciousness from the time of injury indicates that physical damage to the brain has occurred. This is not amenable to surgery. Unconsciousness followed by recovery indicates that cerebral damage is minimal and, if unconsciousness recurs, it can only be due to some progressive lesion; this must be a haemorrhage, which can be stopped by surgery, and recovery can be anticipated if the operation is performed at an early stage on the same side as the dilated pupil. If the first burr hole does not reveal the haemorrhage, the other side should be explored. The prognosis is always better in children and young adults, which justifies a more aggressive surgical approach in this age group.

Open injuries

Clinical assessment and management are similar in both open and closed head injuries, but the patient with an open head injury will require admission for surgery after the application of a sterile dressing to the wound. Care must be taken not to overlook the importance of the clinical state or to allow one's judgement to be clouded by the more spectacular nature of the open injury. A patient with a gross open lesion may make a good recovery.

X-Ray examination

Discussion of the X-ray examination has deliberately been left until this stage. There is a tendency to rush the patient to the X-Ray Department before adequate clinical assessment has been made. This is due to a failure to appreciate that, except in the open injury, the management of the patient is dictated by the neurological state and not by the X-ray findings. A normal X-ray does not exclude the development or presence of an intracranial haematoma; the presence of a fracture may, however, assist in the later management of the patient.

The patient sent to the X-Ray Department with a head injury should always be accompanied by a nurse, who should make regular observations about the patient's level of consciousness, the size and reaction of the pupils, the pulse and respiratory rates and the blood pressure.

Ideally, four views of the skull are necessary, but this may be difficult in a restless patient (*Figure 4.2*).

When the pictures suggest a depressed fracture is present, tangential views across the fracture are necessary to show the extent of the depression. These views should always be taken in open fractures to exclude the presence of inwardly displaced fragments of bone or foreign matter.

Linear fractures of a varying degree of complexity are the commonest finding. When a fracture runs across the meningeal grooves in the temporal region, there may be damage to one of the meningeal vessels and a close watch should be kept on the patient for the early signs of an extradural haemorrhage. When present, the first burr hole should be made in that area.

Separation of the suture lines indicates that considerable force has been applied to the skull. It occurs more often in the younger age groups; in the older age groups very considerable violence is necessary to produce this lesion.

A search should always be made for the pineal body; this is calcified in about 30 per cent of adults. Measurements should be made with a ruler between the outer table of the skull on each side and the pineal

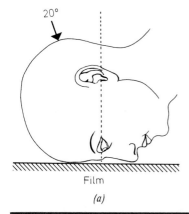

20°

Film

(a)

Figure 4.2. (a) Apart from right and left lateral views, a P-A view with the tube inclined at 20° inferiorly is used to show the frontal and parietal bones. (b) No fracture can be seen in this P-A view of the skull. (c) A Towne's view (A-P with the tube inclined 30° inferiorly) of the same patient shows a linear fracture of the left occipital bone

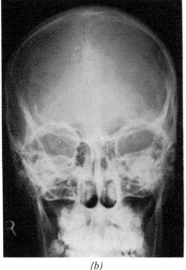

(b)

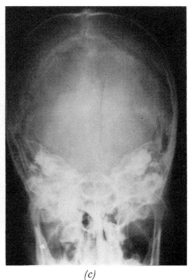

(c)

body to assess if a shift has occured (*Figure 4.3*).When this shift is present, it indicates displacement of the brain and the cause, which is usually a haemorrhage, requires treatment.

Patients who suffer a fracture through the cribriform area of the skull and who later have cerebrospinal rhinorrhoea, may develop a traumatic aerocoele. This is a condition in which a saccular distension of the frontal lobes arises, resulting from a fistula between the frontal lobe and the nasal cavity. An operation to close the hole in the dura and remove the fistulous track results in a satisfactory cure.

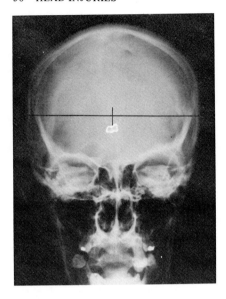

Figure 4.3. Measurements to be made to assess pineal displacement. No shift was present in this patient

Children

The natural history of a head injury is modified in children. Young children and babies can sustain large fractures of the skull with minimal disturbance to their general condition. After a blow or a fall, which may not cause any loss of consciousness, a soft doughy swelling develops on the head which, when discovered by the parents, results in a rapid visit to the doctor or the hospital. X-Ray examination reveals a linear fracture.

The child with a recent fracture should be admitted for observation but, as many of these cases are brought to the hospital two or three days after the injury, there is little point in admitting the child, who can be allowed home after appropriate advice and instructions have been given to the parents, and the General Practitioner has been notified about the injury to his patient.

Children, after a blow on the head, even in the absence of a fracture, may develop generalized convulsions. These are very alarming to the parents and a cause of concern to the young doctor. If neurological examination is otherwise normal, intravenous diazepam should be used to control the attack, which should not be allowed to continue or permanent cerebral damage may occur. Children with more extensive cerebral damage can often be recognized, as they are wheeled into the department, by a high-pitched whining type of cry − the so-called meningeal cry. They tend to be restless and confused and resent examination. Management follows the standard pattern, but care must be taken not to leave the child alone in case he should fall off the trolley. Gentle restraint by wrapping the child up in a blanket is helpful, but the presence of a nurse is essential. Apart from fits, children are prone to vomit after relatively minor head injuries. This can usually be anticipated by their pallor. No child showing this sign should be allowed home without an hour or two being spent under observation. Vomiting after a head injury should be regarded as an indication to admit the child for observation.

SUBDURAL HAEMATOMA

Subdural haematomas are commonest in young children and the elderly. The acute subdural haemorrhage in an elderly patient presents in a similar manner to the acute extradural haemorrhage in younger persons and can only be distinguished from it by operation.

In contrast, the classical subdural, in both age groups, is a quieter, less spectacular condition than an extradural haemorrhage. In both age groups it usually occurs after a relatively minor injury and is due to rupture of a fine bridging vein between the surface of the brain and the meninges caused by an acceleration—deceleration strain on the head. In children this follows shaking or accidental jerks of the head (rarely after fractures or blood clotting disorders) and is uncommon after the age of 3.

In the elderly, a blow caused by banging the top of the head on a shelf or cupboard door when straightening up from a stooping position is sufficient to produce the condition. There may be no loss of consciousness and the patient may not remember the incident. Such patients are unlikely to present in the A & E Department, but the junior doctor should be aware of the possibility of this condition developing after minor trauma in elderly persons.

A young child can present with varying degrees of alteration in consciousness. The child may be listless, fretful and may exhibit weakness of one or more limbs. Dilatation and conjugative deviation of the pupils may be present. Ophthalmoscopy may show papilloedema and retinal haemorrhages. The circumference of the skull may be increased, and X-ray examination may show separation of the suture lines. These children should be referred to the Paediatric Department with a view to subdural tapping being performed.

The elderly patient will present with a history of impairment of the mental faculties extending over a few weeks or months (compared to the two or three years which is found in senile cerebral degeneration). The memory shows marked deterioration, there may be confusion and the gait and balance can be disturbed. Examination may show ocular paralysis and papilloedema. X-Ray examination may show a pineal shift away from the side of the lesion but, if the haemorrhage is bilateral, there will be no change in its position. The diagnosis can be confirmed by cerebral angiography, but axial tomography may clarify the diagnosis of this type of intracranial haemorrhage.

Medical advice may be required to exclude conditions of a non-surgical nature.

GENERAL MANAGEMENT

Careful attention to the airway is essential in all patients with altered consciousness. Any obstruction of the airway causing hypoxia results in increased cerebral damage and deterioration in the patient's condition. Blood, vomit or other fluid in the upper air passages must be sucked out. If other injuries permit, the recovery position, the oropharyngeal airway and suction should suffice to keep the air passages clear in most patients.

The unresponsive patient, even without foreign matter in the upper air passages, is best treated by the insertion of a cuffed endotracheal tube. These can become blocked by a blood clot or secretion, and tracheal toilet by suction with a soft catheter is necessary.

The patient who shows gradual depression of the respiration is a difficult moral and ethical problem. The use of a mechanical ventilator will maintain an adequate degree of oxygenation for bodily survival, but recovery of the mental faculties in these patients becomes increasingly remote in older patients. The situation is still unresolved; it may be justified to use the ventilator in patients under 25, but over this age the prospects of recovery diminish. The advice of a Consultant Anaesthetist or Surgeon should be sought before deciding to use this apparatus in the older patient.

Beware the head injury patient who needs transfusion. Any patient who shows signs of haemorrhagic shock in the absence of any visible injury (e.g. closed major limb fractures), is bleeding internally. An isolated closed head injury never gives rise to shock. Such a patient is suffering from haemorrhage into the pleural or abdominal cavities or may have sustained a fractured pelvis. This latter injury is frequently seen in elderly persons who are knocked down on the road.

Lacerations

Lacerations of the scalp can bleed profusely; this haemorrhage must always be controlled before a patient leaves the department for any purpose. In most patients the application of a dressing, held in place by a firm bandage, will suffice. When there is profuse haemorrhage from a large bleeding point it must be stopped either by the temporary application of an artery forceps, or by under-running the bleeding point with a stitch, the ends of which should be left long to allow easy removal when the laceration is sutured.

The suture of lacerations follows standard practice. The hair should be clipped and shaved for a distance of 2.5–5.0 cm around the wound. Local anaesthetic should be injected and any devitalized tags of tissue should be excised. Bleeding should be stopped by catgut ligatures and general oozing is dealt with by firm pressure, maintained for 4 minutes. A search is made for foreign bodies, such as glass from car windows. The galea is sutured with catgut and the skin with silk or synthetic material. For a small wound, chromic collagen sutures are useful, because they will be absorbed within 10 days and do not need to be removed.

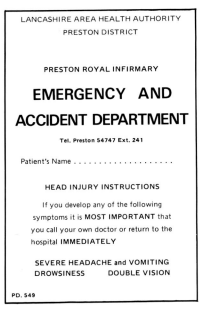

LANCASHIRE AREA HEALTH AUTHORITY
PRESTON DISTRICT

PRESTON ROYAL INFIRMARY

EMERGENCY   AND

ACCIDENT DEPARTMENT

Tel. Preston 54747 Ext. 241

Patient's Name . . . .

HEAD INJURY INSTRUCTIONS

If you develop any of the following symptoms it is MOST IMPORTANT that you call your own doctor or return to the hospital IMMEDIATELY

SEVERE HEADACHE and VOMITING
DROWSINESS   DOUBLE VISION

PD. 549

Figure 4.4.   A head injury card

If the haemorrhage has been well controlled, a dressing is unnecessary. If it is felt that oozing may occur, a dressing held in place by a firm bandage may be used for 24 hours, after which the wound should be left open. Plastic sprays, adhesive strapping and adhesive dressings should not be used. They make suture removal difficult, they will be painful to remove and they serve no useful therapeutic function.

Tetanus prophylaxis is carried out and, if necessary, antibiotics are prescribed for the patient before he leaves the department. Linear wounds should not require antibiotic cover, but the contused wound or the wound which has been contaminated by road dirt is an indication for the use of systemic antibiotics.

All patients with head injuries and the parents or guardians in the case of children who are going home should be advised about the conditions which necessitate an urgent return to the hospital. Provided the patient can read, this is best achieved by giving them a head injury card (*Figure 4.4*).

Non-absorbable sutures are normally removed on the fifth day. Healing of the scalp, because of its good blood supply, is rapid and, if the initial suturing has been properly carried out, infection or other complications should not occur. If healing is slow, alternate sutures may be removed and the patient seen again in 3 days.

5

Injuries to the Face

The facial skeleton is particularly vulnerable to trauma and injuries of the area form an important part of the work in any department. They occur in all age groups and vary between minor, undisplaced fractures of the nose to major disruptions of the facial skeleton which may threaten the life of the victim. If the consequences of deformity are to be avoided, early treatment is essential; unfortunately, this is one of the few areas of the body where major injuries are sometimes missed, even by experienced personnel. This arises from three causes:

1. Failing to obtain an accurate history of the accident.
2. Swelling develops very rapidly and in many cases, by the time the patient reaches hospital, the deformity is concealed and only becomes visible again when the swelling subsides.
3. Inexperience resulting in a failure to recognize that a major injury is present.

When a major facial injury is present in a patient suffering from multiple injuries, the facial injury may require priority in treatment if the patient is to survive. In other cases there may be little urgency when it is an isolated lesion but, because the X-rays are difficult to interpret, it is always advisable to seek the advice of an expert if there is any doubt as to the action to be taken.

FRACTURES OF THE NOSE

The incidence of this injury rises on Saturday nights after the public houses close and the street brawls commence. Nevertheless, any blow to the nose may result in a fracture, but this does not necessarily imply that treatment is necessary.

The deformity of a nasal fracture is characteristic, with deviation to the right or left sides. Unfortunately, swelling may completely mask the

35

altered contour and, because this may have occurred by the time the patient has reached hospital, confirmation of the displacement will not be possible for 5 days, by which time the swelling will have subsided and the deformity will be visible. The nose will be tender, epistaxis of a varying degree will usually be present and, in a severe case, mobility of the bones can be felt by light finger pressure.

X-Ray examination, though essential, can be deferred until the following morning if the patient arrives when the X-Ray Department is only open for the examination of major injuries. The films will show whether or not a fracture has been sustained, but they will not enable the presence of deformity to be established. When a deformity is recognized at the time of the initial visit, the patient should be referred to the Ear, Nose and Throat Department for corrective surgery. This is necessary primarily to correct the deformity and, particularly in females, for cosmetic reasons. It is also necessary to ensure that deviation of the nasal septum does not develop. (Some men may refuse treatment and accept the deformity. A note must always be made to this effect on the records.)

When the nose is very swollen and a fracture is present, the patient should be reviewed in 5 days, by which time the swelling should have resolved sufficiently to assess whether referral is necessary. Minor degrees of deformity are difficult to assess, and even the patient, when asked to look at his or her nose in a mirror, may not be able to indicate whether or not it is out of shape. If in doubt, the opinion of an ear, nose and throat surgeon should be obtained.

If surgical treatment is not required, apart from warning the patient not to blow his nose, no specific measures are necessary.

FRACTURES OF THE ZYGOMA

These injuries are usually unilateral; the bilateral variety occurs as part of the complex of maxillary injuries. Any blow on the cheek can give rise to a fracture and the injury may be sustained in a fight, by contact with a knee in rugby, a head in football or a cricket ball which the victim fails to catch.

The untreated fracture may have four unpleasant consequences for the patient:

1. A cosmetic deformity caused by depression of the prominence of the cheek.
2. A crippling vertical diplopia caused by depression of the floor of the orbit, herniation of the peri-ocular fat and subsequent fibrosis and adhesions around the inferior extra-ocular muscles.

3. Anaesthesia of the cheek, upper lip and inner aspect of the upper lip caused by pressure on the infra-orbital nerve as it emerges from the infra-orbital foramen. (In many cases the patient is unaware of the anaesthesia; but in some it is the presenting symptom.)
4. Interference with free mobility of the mandible when eating, caused by the depressed posterior process of the zygoma impinging on the mandible when biting.

The face should be inspected from the front and from above and behind (*Figure 5.1*). The depression may be clearly visible or it may be masked by swelling and ecchymosis of the eyelids (this is usual in the

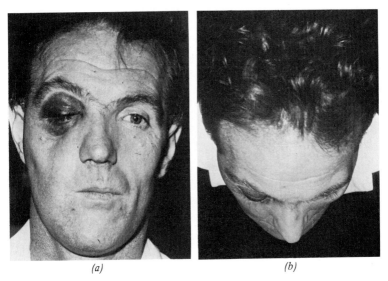

(a)   *(b)*

Figure 5.1.   (a) Depressed fracture of right zygoma caused by cricket ball. (b) The same patient seen from above, showing the difference between the outline of the zygomic arch on each side

Saturday night brawl). The lower margin of the orbit should be gently palpated; a step may be felt near the medial corner. Anaesthesia of the cheek adjacent to the alae nasi and upper lip, and the inner aspect of the upper lip and the adjacent gum should be tested by gentle stroking with a finger. A finger inserted gently under the upper lip towards the orbit may be able to feel a deformity.

The patient should be asked to open and close the jaw and to bite the teeth together; this may reveal impingement caused by depression of the posterior process (*Figure 5.2*). Depression of the main body of the bone does not usually interfere with movement of the mandible. The extent of the injury can only be assessed by X-ray examination in special positions.

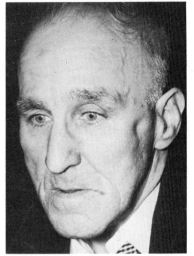

Figure 5.2. Depression caused by fracture of posterior process of zygoma

The X-rays are very difficult for inexperienced Casualty Officers to interpret. The presence of an opaque antrum is strongly suggestive of a fracture of the zygoma but, when in doubt, the opinion of a maxillo-facial surgeon should be sought. If the referral of a depressed fracture is delayed more than 3 days, correction can be difficult and it may not be possible to obtain complete reposition of the bone. The effects mentioned earlier may be permanent and, in particular, vertical diplopia will cause a major disability.

Some undisplaced fractures do have associated infra-orbital anaes-thesia. While no treatment (apart from avoiding blowing of the nose if epistaxis has occurred) is required for these injuries, the patient should be warned that recovery from the anaesthesia may take some months. Similarly, gradual recovery occurs if anaesthesia has resulted from direct trauma to the nerve without any fracture being present.

ORBITAL EMPHYSEMA

Occasionally patients may be seen who complain that, following blowing their nose, their eyelids become swollen. On examination, the eyelids are swollen and surgical emphysema is present in the tissue. The cause

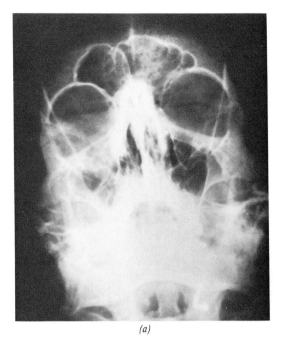

(a)

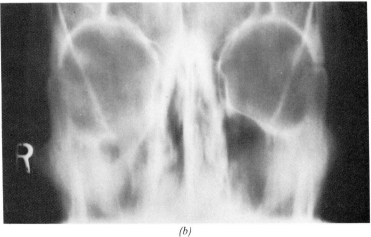

(b)

Figure 5.3. *(a) Apparently undisplaced fracture of right zygoma. There is no depression of the orbital margin, but the lower cortex of the floor of the orbit/roof of antrum is disrupted in a downward direction and encroaches into the body of the antrum. (b) Tomograms confirm the diagnosis of a blow-out fracture*

is a rupture of the epithelial lining of one of the nasal sinuses, with expulsion of air into the medial aspect of the eyelids. In some patients bubbles of air can be seen entrapped in the conjunctiva. No treatment is required, apart from reassurance and the avoidance of nose blowing.

BLOW-OUT FRACTURES OF THE ORBIT

These injuries have only been recognized comparatively recently. They are caused by a blow to the cheek causing a fracture of the floor of the orbit. At the time of the injury the increased orbital pressure drives the orbital contents through the fracture. When the orbital pressure drops, the fracture closes, trapping the orbital contents. The orbital fat, the inferior oblique and the inferior rectus muscles may be caught in the fracture and, if they are not released within a short period, they will become oedematous and fibrosed. Normal function is impossible and vertical diplopia develops from the time of injury. This can be a crippling disability and, when it is suspected, the patient should be referred immediately to the Maxillo-Facial Unit.

Any patient who has sustained a blow to the cheek should be tested for diplopia when looking upwards to the right and to the left. Diplopia on looking to the side away from the injury suggests tethering of the infra-orbital muscles. A fracture may be visible on the X-rays, which may also show the typical pear drop appearance in the lower orbital margin. Tomograms will confirm the diagnosis (*Figure 5.3*).

FRACTURES OF THE MAXILLA

These fractures are frequently missed, particularly when the patient is suffering from other major injuries. This happens when an adequate history is not taken and a perfunctory examination is carried out without realizing that a swollen face, without apparent deformity, can conceal a major and life endangering injury. Such fractures are found after road traffic and sporting accidents and after a brawl where the boot has been used as a weapon.

The various fractures have been classified into the Le Forte types I, II and III. This classification is of little interest to the Casualty Officer compared to the importance of realizing that these are very serious injuries with an appreciable risk to the life of the patient. This arises from three principal causes:

1. The maxilla, which may be completely detached from the base of the skull, can be extremely mobile. If the patient lies in the supine

position, the maxilla will displace posteriorly and occlude the pharynx.

2. Profuse bleeding occurs from the fracture surfaces. This may produce laryngeal obstruction, especially if the patient is in the supine position. The danger will be increased if the mandible is fractured, because the patient will be unable to clear his mouth and throat without assistance, and the tongue may fall back and occlude the larynx.

3. Cerebrospinal fluid leak is a common occurrence in these injuries. It cannot be recognized in the acute stage due to bleeding from the nose and mouth and is usually diagnosed a few days after the injury when the haemorrhage and oedema have subsided.

In a patient who has been assaulted there is an added risk if the neck has been kicked. Oedema of the laryngeal area may develop. This will be greatly increased if the hyoid bone is fractured and may be sufficient to cause a complete obstruction of the larynx.

TREATMENT

Treatment of the injury starts at the scene of the incident. It is imperative that a clear airway be maintained and at no time should the patient be left unattended in case obstruction should develop.

First Aid

The safest position in which to transport the conscious patient is sitting up with the forehead supported on the hands and inclined slightly forwards. Gravity ensures that the maxilla falls away from the posterior pharyngeal wall and the blood flows away from the larynx. Whenever the patient's condition permits, this method should be adopted. If this is not practical either because of the presence of shock or other injuries, the patient should be transported in the recovery position. Suction should be used to remove the blood and any other secretions present in the mouth.

If the patient is unconscious, without other injuries, the recovery position should be used. A pharyngeal airway may be inserted if available (a conscious patient will not tolerate the insertion of an airway) and suction will assist in the removal of the blood. It should be remembered that the insertion of an airway does not guarantee freedom of respiration. The blood may clot in the airway and obstructions can develop suddenly, even when everything is apparently under control.

Certain injuries, e.g. a fractured femur, may prevent the recovery position being used. In these cases a pillow should be placed under one shoulder and the head turned to the opposite side. Suction and an airway should be used when available.

Diagnosis

On arrival at hospital the possibility of a fractured maxilla should be considered whenever a patient arrives with a history of a blow to the face. The classical description given to faces which show marked depression of the central segment is 'dish face' (*Figure 5.4*), but oedema

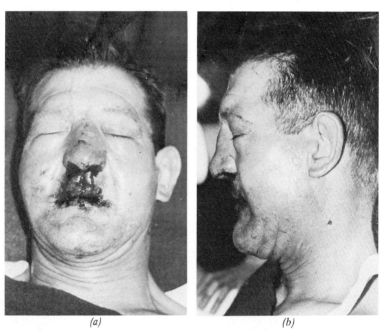

(a)   (b)

Figure 5.4.   (a) and (b) A-P and lateral views of a patient exhibiting the classical 'dish face' deformity. Note absence of swelling

may completely mask the sunken appearance caused by the displacement and it is these cases which may be missed, even when marked displacement is present (*Figure 5.5*). Fractures of the zygoma, which are always present in these injuries, may be seen with ease but can sometimes be masked by the swelling (*Figure 5.6*).

43

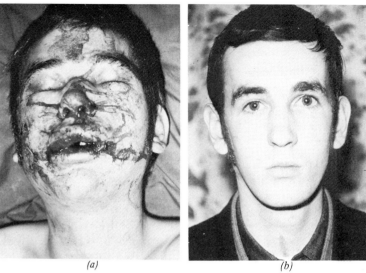

(a)   (b)

Figure 5.5. (a) This patient sustained a middle third fracture of the face associated with a fractured mandible. Note concealment of classical deformity by swelling and the presence of impressions of a rubber-soled shoe on his neck and left cheek. (b) The same patient after 6 months. The degree of swelling present initially can be assessed by reference to (a)

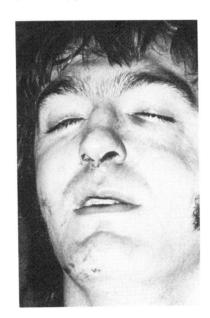

Figure 5.6. Depressed fracture of left zygoma seen from below. This fracture was part of a middle third complex sustained while playing rugby

Examination involves inspection from the front and from above. This latter position may enable fractures of the zygomata to be seen more clearly, and may confirm depression of the orbital margin. Inspection and palpation may confirm the presence of a fractured nose. Damage may be caused to the teeth of the upper jaw, which may be missing, displaced or still attached to mobile segments of the alveolar margin. Mal-occlusion of the teeth will be noticeable.

A finger inserted (gently) into the mouth may enable fractures of the maxilla or zygomata to be palpated and final proof of the injury can be obtained by applying gentle forward traction of the maxilla with the thumb on the outer surface of the upper gum and the index finger on the hard palate. The forward displacement of the maxilla cannot be overlooked, but this manoeuvre should not be repeated unnecessarily; movement of the fracture can cause an increase of the haemorrhage into the mouth or nose, which will increase the problems of management. On many occasions these fractures are associated with fractures of the mandible. This associated injury increases the hazard to the patient but does not demand a greater degree of supervision and attention, since these patients already need the maximal degree of care.

Management

Management in the department involves positioning, as described above, to ensure the integrity of the airway. If the patient is unconscious, an attempt may be made to pass a cuffed endotracheal tube. This is an extremely difficult undertaking in these patients due to the amount of blood that may be present and, when the patient's airway is difficult to control and intubation is considered an urgent matter, the assistance of an experienced anaesthetist should be requested. However much care is given to the airway by positioning the patient, suction to clear the pharynx and the use of an airway, many of these patients show a persisting minor degree of airway obstruction. The breathing is noisy and the patient is restless. Sedative drugs which depress the breathing are absolutely contra-indicated at this stage; intubation cannot be carried out on the conscious or unconscious and non-relaxed patient and the administration of a general anaesthetic on the unprepared patient is a hazardous undertaking.

The ideal treatment for patients who show airway obstruction and who cannot be given a general anaesthetic is a tracheostomy and the insertion of a cuffed tracheostomy tube. This operation, which may have to be carried out under a local anaesthetic, possibly on a restless patient, is technically extremely difficult and it is not advisable for an inexperienced surgeon to attempt it. An experienced ear, nose and throat surgeon should be asked for help in the initial management of the patient, who should not be removed from the department until the airway is under control.

When a major degree of pharyngeal haemorrhage persists, a blood transfusion should be commenced and arrangements made for further supplies to be available later. Even in the absence of other injuries,

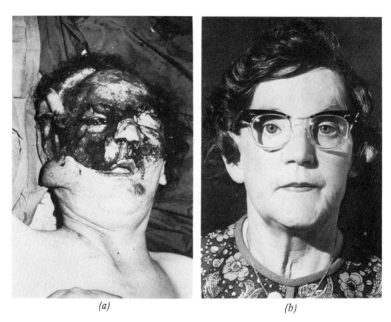

(a)	*(b)*

Figure 5.7.   (a) A gross facial lesion with extensive stripping of the skin, a middle third fracture, and a fracture of the mandible in an elderly patient suffering from rheumatoid arthritis. Even though not associated with other injuries, an injury of this nature carries a very grave risk to the patient's life. Haemorrhage is severe and airway obstruction a constant hazard. (b) The same patient 18 months after the injury. In spite of the major skin damage, skin excision was only required in two minor areas, which are not visible because of her hair. No sloughing of her skin occurred and, after initial tracheostomy and transfusion, her treatment was straightforward

major haemorrhage from the very vascular tissues can give rise to a severe blood loss and it is preferable to anticipate this possibility. Reduction of the fractures, which is necessary before complete control of the bleeding can be obtained, may give rise to further haemorrhage and, when other major injuries are present, the maxillo-facial component must not be overlooked (*Figure 5.7*).

X-Ray examination

X-Ray examination may be required by the maxillo-facial services, but the patient should not be sent for this procedure immediately. The patient will have to be placed in several positions, some of which may cause airway obstruction, and it is dangerous to attempt this investigation unless the integrity of the airway can be guaranteed. It is extremely noticeable that, as soon as the dangers to the airway are removed, if necessary by tracheostomy, much of the patient's restlessness disappears and the subsequent management is greatly simplified. The radiographer will take occipito-mental and lateral views and may wish to take several exposures to demonstrate fully the damage to the facial skeleton. Interpretation of the films is not easy for a relatively inexperienced Casualty Officer and is best left to the experts.

Treatment

Treatment consists in reducing the fracture by manipulation, the fitting of a splint to the upper teeth and the application of traction from the splint to a vertical pillar attached to a cap band around the patient's

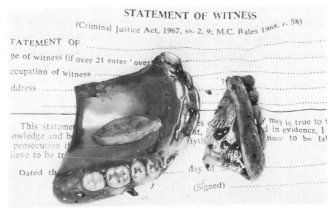

Figure 5.8.   Upper denture brought in by police who were asked to search the patient's car following an accident in which he sustained a middle third fracture

head. In an edentulous patient, the dentures can provide a ready made splint and avoid the delay caused by taking impressions for the manufacture of a suitable splint. If the dentures are brought in with the patient, even if they are broken into several pieces, they can be repaired and provide a splint which will fit the normal configurations of the patient's upper jaw. If the dentures are missing, the ambulance or police services should be requested to search the accident site to see if they can be recovered (*Figure 5.8*). The possibility that missing teeth or pieces of dentures may be lodged in a bronchus should not be overlooked and X-ray examination of the chest should be carried out at the same time as the patient is in the department for X-ray examination of his injuries.

In assaults about the face, the neck is frequently kicked. This may result in soft tissue oedema and possibly fractures of the laryngeal and hyoid cartilages; these injuries will cause swelling and possibly laryngeal obstruction. Breathing will be noisy, the conscious patient restless and distressed and cyanosis will be present. Tracheostomy is urgently needed, particularly when the neck injury is associated the facial and/or mandibular fractures, but it must only be carried out by someone with experience. In these patients it is one of the most difficult of emergency operations and, in unskilled hands, could kill or seriously prejudice the patient's recovery.

FRACTURES OF THE MANDIBLE

The characteristic features of this injury are pain, swelling and difficulty in biting after an injury. The fractures may be unilateral or bilateral and may give rise to mal-occlusion of the teeth. Haemorrhage may also arise from tears of the gum at the site of the fracture (*Figure 5.9*).

Fractures of the horizontal ramus of the mandible present little difficulty in diagnosis, but fractures of the neck or condyle of the mandible, which are frequently bilateral and caused by trauma to the point of the chin, may have relatively few signs or symptoms. This possibility should be remembered in patients who present with only slight tenderness of the temporo-mandibular area. X-Ray examination is necessary to establish the diagnosis and the best views are given by the orthopantograph, usually referred to as an OPG view (*Figure 5.10*). The picture produced by this machine can be regarded as an opened-out picture of the mandible, with each area taken at a right-angle. The initial strangeness on seeing such a view can be overcome by folding the film round into the shape of the mandible.

Patients with fractures of the mandible should be referred to the oral surgeons for treatment. If the fracture is undisplaced, the jaw should be supported with a bandage and the patient advised to eat soft food until he can be seen in the next clinic. If there is any displacement, advice should be obtained from the Specialist Unit before the patient is allowed to leave the hospital.

48

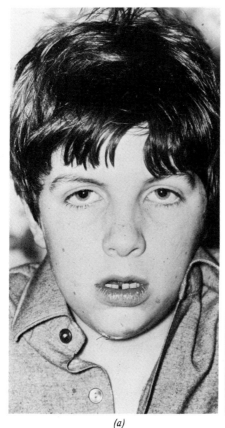

Figure 5.9. (a) Fracture of the mandible sustained in a fall on the point of the chin. The gap between and the step in the level of the teeth is clearly visible. (b) View of teeth showing disturbance in alignment and bleeding from the fracture between the two central incisors

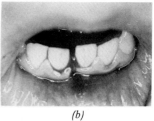

(a) (b)

Figure 5.10. OPG view of mandible showing fracture through the neck of the condyle on the left side

In the conscious patient these injuries do not usually give rise to respiratory embarrassment but, in the unconscious patient, or when there is a major compound lesion (*Figure 5.11*) in either the conscious or unconscious patient there is a risk, which is increased when the facial

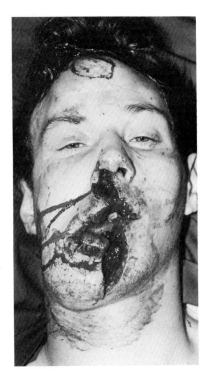

Figure 5.11. Compound fracture of the mandible associated with damage to the teeth of the upper jaw. This patient is at a risk of airway obstruction

bones are also injured, of respiratory obstruction. This must be treated by positioning of the patient, the use of the sucker and airway if the patient is unconscious and, in severe obstruction, intubation may be necessary. This procedure, in these patients, can be extremely difficult and the assistance of an expert should always be obtained if time allows.

DENTAL ABSCESSES

Patients, frequently children, often present in the department with a tender, painful swelling along the side of the jaw which has developed a day or two after a blow (*Figure 5.12*). X-Ray examination does not reveal any bony damage, but inspection of the teeth in the area usually

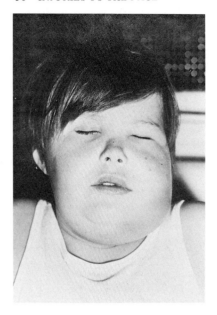

Figure 5.12. Large dental abscess developing 5 days after a minor blow to the left side of the jaw. This was associated with severe caries of two teeth in the adjacent part of the mouth

shows dental caries which is associated with tenderness on percussion with a spatula. The X-ray should be reviewed for evidence of infection around the apex of the root of the carious or tender tooth. Even without X-ray evidence of apical infection, the diagnosis is one of dental abscess.

A course of penicillin should be prescribed and the patient advised to consult a dental practitioner.

SOFT TISSUE INJURIES

The high vascularity of facial tissues ensures that lacerations will heal rapidly. For the same reason, excision of damaged tissues should be minimal. Small tags of skin which, in other areas, would be removed, usually survive. Excision should be confined to tissue which is grossly damaged and heavily contaminated with dirt which cannot be removed in any other manner. Over-enthusiastic removal of damaged tissues may cause a soft tissue deformity which will make later repair more difficult and it is important not to complicate later reconstruction by an injudicious technique after the initial injury.

The cosmetic aspects of facial wounds, particularly in females of all ages, must never be forgotten. Whenever it is thought that the injury will give rise to a significant degree of disfigurement – which will vary with the age of the patient — advice should always be obtained from the Plastic Surgery Unit before commencing repair of the laceration. Plastic surgeons possess no skills which are not available to the junior doctor. Their apparently remarkable results are obtained solely by taking time with careful attention to detail, coupled with gentle handling of the tissues.

The instruments used for suture should be designed for the purpose. The use of instruments suitable for abdominal or orthopaedic surgery is inappropriate for the gentle handling of damaged facial tissues. The wound edges should be handled with skin hooks or fine dissecting forceps. Artery forceps should never be applied to the skin edges and scissors should be sharp, with an undamaged cutting edge. Haematoma formation must be avoided by ensuring that bleeding has stopped before suturing is commenced. Pressure or ligation of the bleeding points will ensure a dry wound.

Except in small wounds, the subcutaneous tissues should be sutured with fine catgut on an atraumatic needle. This avoids tension being placed on the skin sutures, which then serve only to hold the wound edges in apposition. This enables very fine suture material (5/0 or 6/0 on atraumatic needles) to be used and allows removal after 2 or 3 days. Many wounds can be sutured under local anaesthetic, which does distend the tissues and can make re-alignment of the edges more difficult. This can be avoided by the use of hyaluronidase (1500 units) in 10 ml of the local anaesthetic. This will reduce the period of anaesthesia and a further infiltration may be necessary in part of the wound if repair has not been completed in time.

The eyebrows should never be shaved. This would destroy an important re-alignment mark needed during the repair of the laceration. Wounds of the eyelids should be referred to the Ophthalmic Department. Repair of the edges of these structures is technically difficult and, in the medial third, the laceration may have damaged the nasolacrimal duct.

Wounds of the edges of the lips need careful repositioning of the pink margin if significant cosmetic disability is to be avoided. In through and through wounds of the lips, the muscle and mucosa should be repaired with catgut. Not infrequently they are caused by the teeth and, if a tooth is damaged, it may be found inside the tissues of the lip. If palpation is not practical because of swelling, X-ray examination using a dental film may be necessary.

After treatment

After suture has been completed, the wound edges should be covered with a thin film of ophthalmic ointment and the wound left exposed.

When the cosmetic aspects are important, the wound should be inspected daily and crusts and clots gently removed from the suture line. It may be possible to remove alternate sutures at 48 hours and the rest a day later. If a small haematoma develops, it should be evacuated after removing one suture.

Plastic sprays make suture removal difficult and painful. Powders cake on the wound and occlusive adhesive dressings ensure that superficial infection will occur. Dressings stick to the wound and may, when removed, cause partial disruption of the suture line. Provided the initial suturing has been carried out with care and the wound edges are in good apposition, the wound will be sealed within a few hours and infection will not occur. Nature is still the doctor's best ally and, if properly supported, can be relied upon to produce a better result than all the magical powders and chemicals produced by the manufacturers.

ABRASIONS

Dirt engrained abrasions should be scrubbed with a firm brush. This procedure is much less painful than might be anticipated and it is usually possible to carry out an adequate removal of the dirt with topical anaesthesia obtained by the use of an anaesthetic jelly. Only rarely, in nervous patients and young children, should general anaesthesia be necessary.

INTRA-ORAL LESIONS

Damage to teeth is a matter for the patient's dental practitioner. If a sharp edge of a fractured tooth causes discomfort, the edge should be smoothed with fine emery paper until dental attention can be given.

Permanent incisor teeth, which have been knocked out, can be re-implanted. The tooth should be placed in normal saline and sent with the patient to the Dental Department. After it is re-inserted in the socket, it is held in place with a cap splint until it has become re-attached. Even though it is dead and will darken after several years, this is preferable to the immediate provision of a denture, especially in young adolescents.

Lacerations of the tongue should be sutured with catgut. The tip can usually be repaired under local anaesthetic, but lacerations of the dorsal aspect may necessitate a general anaesthetic if repair is to be effectual. Children may need a general anaesthetic for suture in either site.

Lacerations of the palate require suture under a general anaesthetic by someone skilled in this form of surgery. If the posterior pharyngeal wall has been damaged, as for example in a fall with a stick or pencil in the mouth, the possibility that the point of the object has traversed the base of the skull and punctured the meninges must be considered. X-Ray examination should be carried out and the patient admitted for observation.

Lacerations of the gums, which retract and expose the alveolar margins, should always be sutured. If the junior doctor does not feel capable of carrying out this procedure, he should seek help from the Dental Unit.

Patients with bleeding tooth sockets after dental extractions should, whenever possible, be referred back to the dentist who carried out the procedure in the first instance. If this is not practical, after removal of the clot, the socket should be packed with a haemostatic gauze or sponge. The patient should apply pressure to the area by biting on an appropriately sized roller bandage. If this does not control the haemorrhage, a collagen mattress suture should be inserted, after packing with haemostatic gauze or sponge, across the cavity between the gum margins on each side of the socket.

Sedation may be required and, if the haemorrhage has been severe, admission overnight may be necessary. In children, when the haemorrhage has been severe and difficult to control, transfusion might be necessary. In these cases the possibility of a bleeding diathesis must be excluded by appropriate laboratory investigations.

6

Eye Emergencies

The care of eye emergencies is an important part of the work of any Accident and Emergency Department. In many cases the treatment needed is beyond the skills of the unit, but the Accident Officer must be aware of those conditions which may present as acute emergencies and which may require urgent specialized management if the patient's vision is not to be jeopardized.

HISTORY

An accurate history is essential. In many cases the diagnosis can be made on the information supplied by the patient and examination serves as confirmation. The mode of onset of the presenting symptoms is important; a sudden pain coming on, for example, when grinding metal, suggests a foreign body. Itching suggests an allergic condition — has there been any recent change in the make of cosmetics used by the patient? Sudden loss of vision suggests arterial disturbances. Gradual loss of vision, possibly associated with pain, suggests glaucoma.

EXAMINATION

The eyes should be examined from the front. Adult patients can sit; children, who are usually co-operative if a parent is allowed to hold their hand, are easiest to examine if they lie on an examination couch, but sedation or a general anaesthetic may be necessary in an urgent situation. The examiner should stand or sit on the same side of the patient as the injured eye.

A suitable lamp, giving a well focussed, cool beam is essential and a binocular magnifier with a headband and which fits over spectacles is also essential. Practice is necessary to acquire familiarity with the apparatus.

Visual acuity should be assessed. This is essential, even if only crude methods are used. When simple methods, such as reading a book or a newspaper, suggest impairment, then test type should be used. All layers of the eye should be inspected and the shape and reactions of the pupils noted. Ophthalmoscopy is carried out when there are indications, such as disturbances in visual acuity, that there may be disturbances in the function of the posterior ocular structures.

The cornea should always be stained when the history or examination suggests that the epithelial covering may be damaged. A drop of fluorescein is placed in the eye or the impregnated end of a paper strip is placed in the lower conjunctival sac for a few seconds, after which the eye is washed out with normal saline drops. The fluorescein stains corneal defects a bright green, which can be seen very clearly in a blue light or in a narrow beam of well focussed light directed obliquely across the cornea.

If the patient is sitting in a chair, treatment is best carried out by the examiner standing behind the chair. The patient is asked to fix both eyes on a spot in front of him. The use of a special chair, the back of which can be dropped and which carries a head rest, is of considerable help in avoiding extension of the head or neck. This procedure is uncomfortable and can make the patient faint. If the patient is lying on a couch, the examiner should sit at the top of the couch.

LACERATIONS

The treatment of lacerations around the eye follows normal practice. In all but the smaller wound, local anaesthetic should be used. The finest atraumatic suture material should be used and accurate skin apposition, without distortion of the tissue, obtained. The vascularity of the tissue makes excision of small skin tags unnecessary. When there is tissue loss, the patient should be referred to a plastic surgeon.

The eyebrows should never be shaved; this makes it difficult to re-suture the skin with the necessary accuracy and may cause a permanent distortion of the eyebrow. When the wound is above the eyebrow and involves the underlying muscles, these should be sutured with fine catgut to avoid subsequent drooping of the eyebrow. Wounds which involve the edges of the eyelids should be referred to the Ophthalmic Department for repair. This is especially important in those which involve the medial margins of the lids where damage to the lacrimal canaliculi may be present.

CONTUSIONS

Black eyes are common injuries, especially on Saturday nights. The degree of swelling is frequently large enough to make inspection of the eye a difficult task, but whenever possible it should always be inspected for evidence of corneal damage or haemorrhage into the anterior chamber. If possible, the vision should be assessed.

It is usually impossible to feel the lower margin of the orbit, and X-ray examination will be necessary to exclude a fracture of the zygoma or a 'blow-out' fracture of the floor of the orbit. This important complication may give rise to diplopia due to trapping of the inferior rectus and inferior oblique eye muscles in the fracture; this was discussed further in Chapter 5.

If it is impossible to assess diplopia at the time of the injury, the patient, in the absence of X-ray evidence, should be re-examined after 5 or 6 days by which time the swelling will have subsided. The presence of a fracture or diplopia is an indication for the referral of the patient to the Maxillo-Facial Department. The uncomplicated case should be treated by the twice daily application of chloramphenicol eye ointment to prevent the eyelids sticking together.

Small residual localized haematoma usually absorb. Those which fail to do so may resolve after the injection of 1500 units of hyalase into the centre of the haematoma. Incision and evacuation of the clot should only be undertaken if the haematoma is relatively large, firm and likely to take a prolonged period before it finally resolves.

FOREIGN BODIES

Intra-ocular

Intra-ocular foreign bodies should be suspected if the history suggests that the object had a high velocity when it hit the eye. The use of a hammer and chisel, turning metal on a lathe or drilling metal with high-speed drills are all situations which can cause intra-ocular foreign bodies and, even if there is no external evidence of injury, X-ray and ophthalmoscopic examination are essential with this type of history. Even if all the findings are negative, if the doctor still feels that there is a reasonable probability of an intra-ocular foreign body being present, he should refer the patient to the Ophthalmic Department.

Subtarsal

The patient who presents at the door of the department with a handkerchief pressed to the eye and with a history that something blew in the eye a few minutes previously will probably be suffering from a subtarsal foreign body. The eye looks irritable, blinking is painful but no foreign body can be seen.

The upper lid must be everted to show the foreign body. This is easier to perform in the elderly, whose tissues are laxer, than in young

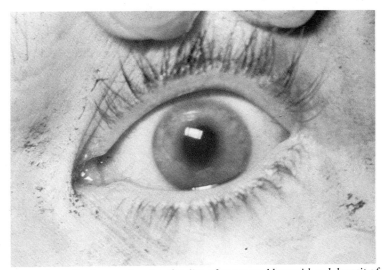

Figure 6.1.   Hyphaema, showing clouding of cornea and brownish red deposit of blood around the lower rim of the cornea. The iris is also obscured by blood in the anterior chamber

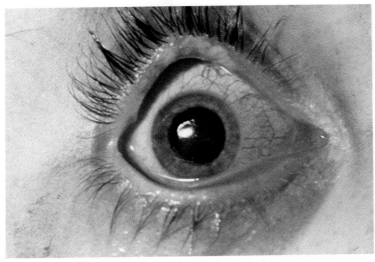

Figure 6.3.   A large central defect of the cornea stained with fluorescein. This injury was caused by a chemical burn

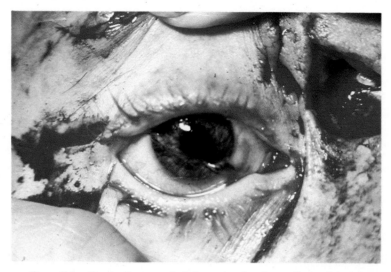

Figure 6.4. *Penetrating wound of the cornea showing prolapse of the iris*

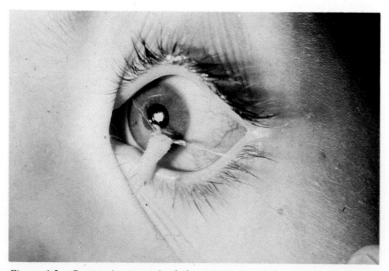

Figure 6.5. *Penetrating wound of the cornea caused by misadventure when fishing. This caused problems with First Aid because pressure, which would be caused if a pad and bandage were used, was inadvisable. The problem was resolved by lightly strapping the eyelids together, using adhesive suture strips, to prevent blinking*

adults. It is carried out by asking the patient to look downwards while the eyelashes are gently held and pulled downwards initially and then forwards and upwards around the upper margin of the tarsal plate, which is depressed either by a finger, a matchstick or a glass rod. The foreign body is removed by wiping with a moistened (saline) pledget or cotton wool wrapped around a wooden spill.

Fluorescein staining will show fine linear abrasions.

After the removal of the foreign body, chloramphenicol eye ointment is applied. An eye pad is used only if local anaesthetic has been necessary to overcome spasm of the eyelids which has prevented eversion of the upper lid.

Conjunctival

Small foreign bodies on the conjunctiva, which cannot be wiped off, can be left. Any attempt at removal causes a haemorrhage into the surrounding tissues, which makes removal completely impossible. Large foreign bodies should be removed in the Ophthalmic Department.

Corneal

While these are generally painful, it is by no means infrequent for patients to report to the department with only minor discomfort from a foreign body which has clearly been present for 2 or 3 days.

It is important that the patient, whether sitting or lying down, should be relaxed during removal of the foreign body. He should be asked to fix both eyes on a point straight ahead and allowed to close the eyes at intervals during the removal to prevent drying of the cornea and to allow the muscles to relax.

Local anaesthetic is essential to remove any foreign body embedded in the cornea. Two or three drops of 1 per cent amethocaine should be given into the lower conjunctiva twice at half-minute intervals, the patient being allowed to blink after each instillation. A binocular loupe fixed to a headband is essential, and a lamp designed for the purpose should be used. Ordinary bulbs in reflectors are very hot and uncomfortable to the patient. If the foreign body has only been *in situ* for a short while, it may be possible to remove it with a cotton wool bud (cotton wool twisted around the end of an orange stick) moistened with local anaesthetic or saline; if it does not detach easily, removal should be continued with the point of a 38 x 0.8 mm hypodermic needle. The doctor should stand behind or above the patient's head, depending on whether the patient is sitting or lying down. The right hand of a right-handed operator should be steadied on the forehead, while the left hand gently parts the eyelids. The needle should be held at an oblique angle to the cornea to avoid impaling the tissues if the patient should move the eye suddenly. The foreign body is removed with the point of the needle and, if it becomes loose and lies on the cornea or lower conjunctiva, it should be wiped away with a moistened cotton wool bud. If it is deeply embedded and cannot be removed without causing further damage, the attempt should be abandoned and the patient referred to the Ophthalmic Department for further treatment.

Rust rings remaining after removal of the foreign body should be left for 3 or 4 days; after this time they are easily removed with the point of a needle. They can also be treated with a chelating agent. Desferrioxamine eye drops used 3 times a day for 4 days may avoid the necessity for further active measures. Unfortunately the drops (*see* Appendix III) have to be made up freshly for each patient, should be kept in a refrigerator and have a limited life. These factors limit the general use of this agent but, in patients who have difficulty in relaxing the eyelid or in whom further active measures may be difficult or inadvisable, consideration should be given to its use.

After removal of the foreign body, chloramphenicol ointment should be inserted and an eye pad applied. With a superficial foreign body the pad can be removed after 4 hours, but when a large crater has been left, healing will be quicker if the pad is kept on for a few days and eye ointment is inserted twice a day. If the eye is very injected or painful, one drop of 1 per cent atropine should be instilled. This should not be used without warning the patient that the vision, particularly for reading, will be disturbed for up to 2 weeks and that bright lights will cause discomfort for a shorter period. It is essential that the disability is sufficient to justify these disturbances to the patient's vision; furthermore, the use of a powerful mydriatic in elderly patients may give rise to acute glaucoma and it is wiser for the Accident Officer to restrict its use to patients under 40 years of age.

CORNEAL ABRASIONS

These are frequently caused by children scratching their mother's eyes, by twigs when gardeners are cutting hedges or during the initial stages of wearing contact lenses when the patient attempts to wear the appliances for a longer time than the eye will tolerate. Eyes exposed to a blast of high pressure from a compressed air line may exhibit foreign bodies and multiple abrasions or generalized fine central abrasions.

Eyes must be stained to demonstrate abrasions. If no foreign body can be seen, an abrasion is frequently present. The history of both conditions is similar and staining is the only method which will allow identification of a pin-head size epithelial defect. Treatment is similar to that used after the removal of a foreign body. Healing is normally rapid, but if it is delayed or followed by marked injection, the patient should be referred to the Ophthalmic Unit. If pain is a major complaint, atropine should be used in the same way that it is used after the removal of a foreign body.

Contact lenses should not be handled by the doctor. They are expensive, easy to lose and are best handled by the patient. If the patient does not possess a suitable container, then it is wise to ask the patient if one provided by the department is suitable. Once such a lens is lost, it is unlikely to be found again and unnecessary acrimony is easy to avoid by judicious forethought.

FLASH BURNS

A superficial keratitis caused by exposure to ultra-violet light is common in welders and is occasionally seen in persons who do not wear goggles when using a 'sun-ray' lamp at home. The condition comes on a few hours after exposure and causes pain, lacrimation and photophobia. Fine superficial pin-point staining may be seen after using fluorescein.

Pain, which may be severe, can be relieved by local anaesthetic drops. Treatment consists of applying chloramphenicol eye ointment followed by an eye pad, held in place by a crêpe bandage. If both eyes are affected a pad and bandage should be applied to both eyes. The patient should be advised to rest in bed and report back to the hospital the following morning, by which time the majority of symptoms should have resolved. Sedatives may be necessary for the first few hours.

HYPHAEMA

Haemorrhage, visible in the anterior chamber of the eye, occurs after direct injury and varies from a slight brownish red deposit around the lower rim of the cornea to a marked and obvious haemorrhage occupying the whole of the anterior chamber (*Figure 6.1, see* plate section facing page 56). The only treatment for this condition is rest, and once it has been diagnosed the patient should be placed on a trolley and a pad and bandage applied to both eyes. Arrangements should be made for the patient to be admitted. Except in severe cases, the condition usually resolves quickly, but glaucoma and fresh haemorrhage may develop after a few days and skilled observation is necessary to detect the onset of these complications.

BURNS

Thermal lesions

Thermal lesions of the eye are commonly found in association with similar lesions of the face. While the patient is in the department, drying of the cornea may be prevented by covering the eye with a single sheet

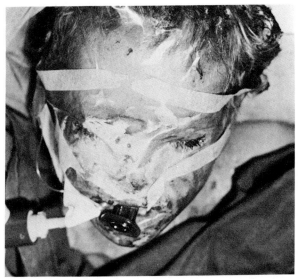

Figure 6.2. A child with severe burns of face and both eyes, showing polythene sheet being used to prevent drying of the cornea

of thin polythene, held in place by adhesive strapping (*Figure 6.2*). These patients should always be referred for an ophthalmic opinion, even if the Plastic Surgery Unit is also involved. It is preferable not to apply ointment before the patient is seen by the Eye Department in order to avoid distorting the appearance of the cornea and making the area slippery and difficult to handle.

Chemical burns

These usually arise from industrial sources but the 'do-it-yourself' car owner may splash battery acid in his eye and the housewife may splash caustic oven cleanser in her eye.

Injuries due to caustic substances cause much greater damage than those from acids; nevertheless treatment of both groups is similar. If the eyes have not been irrigated before the patient arrives at hospital, the eyes should be immediately irrigated with tap water. If the chemical contamination is severe, the head should be immersed under water and the eyelids forced apart. Subsequently, the eyes should be profusely irrigated with large volumes of normal saline after the instillation of local anaesthetic. This process is simplified by using transfusion bottles and giving sets instead of the old-fashioned undine. Buffer solution* has been helpful for immediate use in both acidic and alkaline burns.

The jet of fluid should be directed on all areas of the eye, using an eyelid retractor under the upper eyelid to allow irrigation of the superior fornix of the conjunctiva. At the conclusion of the irrigation, strips of red and blue litmus paper should be gently applied to the conjunctiva to assess the pH. A marked colour change indicates that the irrigation should be continued.

Staining may reveal corneal damage (*Figure 6.3, see* plate section facing page 56) and, if this is more than minimal, the patient should be referred to the Eye Department.

Lime

When the eye has been irrigated before arrival at hospital and no particles of the chemical can be seen, treatment follows the methods indicated above. When the patient arrives with the substance still in the eye, after the instillation of local anaesthetic, the substances should be removed with eye buds, a spud, a needle or forceps. Irrigation is then carried out and the patient referred to the Eye Department.

The preservation, even of minimal vision, is of extreme importance to the patient, and when both eyes are involved attention should initially be given to the less severely affected side, which will have a better chance of recovery than the more severely affected one.

PENETRATING WOUNDS OF THE CORNEA

These injuries are usually easy to recognize and are frequently associated with prolapse of the uveal tissues. This causes an eccentric or ovoid pupil, associated with a small, dark, prolapsed mass of tissue, the overall appearance being similar to an exclamation mark or a comma (*Figures 6.4* and *6.5, see* plate section facing page 56). The anterior chamber is collapsed and the tension is low due to loss of the aqueous humour. A

See Appendix II

pad and bandage should be lightly applied and the patient referred to the Ophthalmic Department for admission.

LACERATIONS OF THE CONJUNCTIVA

Small lacerations heal rapidly with chloramphenicol eye ointment. If there is any retraction of the conjunctiva, the patient should be referred to the Eye Department for suture.

TETANUS PROPHYLAXIS

This should not be overlooked in open wounds of the eye.

7

Injuries to the Chest and Chest Wall

The greater the degree of force to which a patient is exposed, the greater the probability that admission to hospital will be required. An estimate of the forces to which the patient was exposed is also of considerable help in making a tentative assessment about the possibility of a major thoracic or abdominal injury being present. For example, the patient who falls against the edge of a table is unlikely to develop a haemo-pneumothorax; the driver of a car involved in a collision at 60 mph could well be expected to sustain a major injury for which a deliberate search must be made.

After the history has been obtained, examination of the chest follows a standard routine which does not vary significantly between the fully conscious ambulant patient and the unconscious patient suffering from multiple injuries.

EXAMINATION

The conscious patient must be stripped to the waist and asked to identify the painful area and to describe the nature of the pain. His ability to undress himself, to move about and to position himself for examination should be noted.

The unconscious patient should be stripped and the chest left exposed to allow constant observation.

Inspection

The degree of respiratory distress should be recorded and, if cyanosis is not obvious, the lobes of the ears and the sublungual areas of the fingers should be inspected for minor degrees of colour change. Traumatic asphyxia is easily visible.

Haemoptysis may be found in pulmonary contusion or ruptures of the tracheal and bronchial tracts; large amounts of blood-stained frothy sputum are found in pulmonary oedema.

Both sides of the chest should be inspected for the presence of open wounds (sucking wounds are comparatively rare), bruises or imprinting caused by clothing, safety belts or the central boss (*Figure 7.1*) or rim (*Figure 7.2*) of a steering wheel.

The rate and depth of breathing should be assessed prior to inspecting the respiratory movements, which should be studied initially when the patient is breathing 'normally' and then while taking a deep breath. Most patients with fractured ribs will be unable to make more than a slight effort at deep inspiration before the movement is inhibited by pain.

Areas of diminished respiratory excursion should be noted. This may be localized to one area or it may affect the whole of one side.

Paradoxical respiration should be excluded. Only infrequently is it obvious, being in most cases difficult to see and requiring experience to recognize minor degrees of disturbance in the respiratory rhythm. A badly shocked patient suffering from chest and other injuries may not exhibit paradox during the early stages of resuscitation. This is because the patient is incapable of making sufficient respiratory effort for the paradox to become apparent, and a failure to keep a constant watch on such a patient's breathing during resuscitation can result in major chest lesions being overlooked. Patients who exhibit paradoxical movements over a large area of the chest are dyspnoeic with rapid, shallow breathing and some degree of cyanosis. There is great mental distress associated with the condition; this does not make for equanimity on the part of the doctor, but it is essential to make a careful study of the respiratory movements from the top, the bottom and the sides of the trolley if a full assessment is to be made.

It is easy to define paradox as *a reversal of the normal respiratory movement*, but it is not so simple to recognize this in a restless patient with rapid, shallow breathing. It is best to study the chest as a whole, rather than concentrating the vision on the damaged area. The rhythm of the 'normal' areas should be established, after which the abnormal area should be brought into the field of view. Careful study of the rhythms of both areas will establish whether there is a reversal of the movement in the damaged area. The best analogy that can be given is that it is like listening to a tune in which some of the notes are misplaced. An attempt to recognize paradox in individual respiratory excursions will fail but, if the rhythms are studied, abnormalities will be more easily appreciated. Do not, however, confuse the in-drawing of the lower costal margin, which can be seen in many children or old people suffering from chest infections, with paradoxical movement.

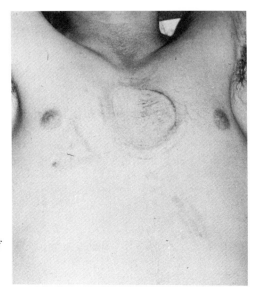

Figure 7.1. Imprint of steering wheel boss

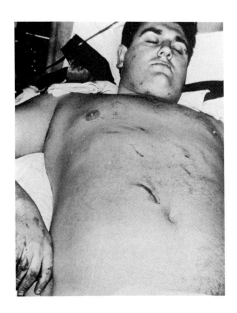

Figure 7.2. Imprints caused by rim of steering wheel

After inspecting the chest, study the abdomen, particularly in the epigastric area, for distension and diminution of movement.

Palpation

Thus far the assessment has been based on talking and looking. The next step involves gentle palpation of the chest.

In the conscious patient start gentle palpation in a pain-free area, gradually moving towards the damaged area. Feel for grating or clicking sensations associated with the breathing. Coarse *râles* may be felt and surgical emphysema will produce a characteristic grating sensation. Large amounts of air in the tissues may give rise to considerable swelling, which may extend to the lower part of the neck or the face. Clicks are present when fractured ribs or costal cartilages move with the respiratory movements.

The flat of each hand should be placed symmetrically on each side of the chest and the movements studied. This manoeuvre may assist in the recognition of paradox. The painful areas should be carefully palpated to establish if the tenderness is located in the ribs or the adjacent soft tissues. The apex beat should be located to assess mediasternal shift, and the suprasternal notch should be palpated for evidence of tracheal displacement. The abdomen is then palpated for evidence of rigidity, tenderness and distension.

Percussion

Percussion is the next step in the examination. This should be carried out as gently as possible, but it may be necessary to turn or raise the patient to examine the back and sides of the chest. If the patient is moved, the opportunity should be taken to auscultate the same areas to avoid an unnecessary disturbance. Hypertympanic areas, when present, indicate a pneumothorax, usually under tension. Dullness is found in collapse of the lung or the presence of fluid.

This procedure should also be carried out on the abdomen. Hypertympanic resonance in the epigastrium suggests gastric dilatation. Dullness in the flanks might indicate intra-abdominal haemorrhage, but to establish this clearly would necessitate testing for shifting of the fluid level. This test is of little value in these cases; it is inaccurate and unjustified and better methods, such as peritoneal lavage, are available.

Auscultation

Auscultation should follow percussion. Much can be learned from a single examination, but repeated examination is essential to avoid missing a progressive intrathoracic lesion. Normal breath sounds, without râles or crepitations, indicate that the underlying lung tissues and the pleural cavity are, at that time, functioning normally.

Clicking sounds may be heard from fractured ribs or along the costo-chondral junctions, where they indicate disruption of the joints, even if no displacement can be felt. Surgical emphysema, small areas of which can be recognized more easily with the stethoscope, gives rise to a grating crepitation, which may conceal the sounds from the deeper areas. Absent breath sounds suggest fluid in the pleural cavity or collapse of the underlying lung.

Bronchial breathing suggests partial collapse of the lung tissues; scattered areas of bronchial breathing suggest intrapulmonary haemorrhage following contusions of the lung. When the breath sounds are very high-pitched and tubular, a tension pneumothorax should be suspected; the coin test may support this contention. This is carried out by placing a coin on the chest wall and striking it with another coin. A clear, high-pitched, bell-like note will be obtained if air under pressure is present in the pleural cavity. When present, rapid relief of the tension using an intravenous cannula may be necessary.

In many cases an accurate picture of the injury can be built up from the examination findings. Nevertheless, X-ray examination should be carried out before treatment is undertaken, provided the delay and necessary movement will not be prejudicial to the patient's recovery.

X-Ray examination

Ambulant patients present no difficulty. A postero-anterior and an oblique view of the side of the lesion are necessary. The area where fractured ribs are suspected should be indicated on the request form to enable the appropriate views to be taken. If it is thought necessary, a specific request should be made for a view of the lung fields, because the increased exposure needed to show rib fractures, together with the necessary positioning for this purpose, does not show pulmonary abnormalities with sufficient clarity to enable minor changes in the lung fields to be recognized at an early stage.

Fractures of the costochondral junctions or of the costal cartilages of the lower ribs cannot be seen on the X-rays. The former can be diagnosed clinically; the latter, apart from the discomfort, are of little significance, and it is doubtful if it is worthwhile X-raying patients whose main complaint is of isolated tenderness of the costal margins.

The patient with an obvious major chest injury presents difficulty, and some patients, whose condition would be adversely affected by movement, may have to have their initial treatment carried out without being X-rayed. Ideally, the films should be taken on a diagnostic X-ray unit with the patient in the erect position in order to show fluid or air in the pleural cavity. If this is not possible, even a slight upward inclination will be of greater help than a film taken with the patient lying flat. Nevertheless, information of a limited, though practical, nature can be obtained from a portable film taken in the Emergency Department with the patient lying flat on the resuscitation trolley (*Figure 7.3*). A film taken in this manner may show surgical emphysema, some fractured

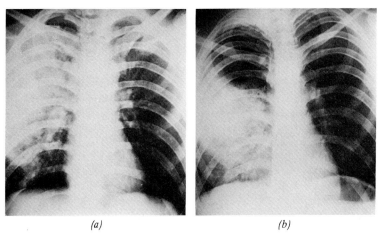

(a)   *(b)*

Figure 7.3.   X-Rays of same patient taken at the same time showing extensive contusion of the right middle lobe. (a) Was taken with the patient flat, and (b) with the patient erect

ribs and alterations in the density of each lung field. It may show a large pneumothorax; a small pneumothorax will not show, nor will any fine details of the lung structures be visible. A large, diffuse area of opacity, obliterating the lung fields, will suggest the presence of a haemothorax which can be confirmed, if necessary, by aspiration; but fluid levels which occur in a haemopneumothorax will not show up. Fluoroscopy and image intensification are costly, but extremely valuable in the resuscitation room. The moving picture can be far more informative than the still photograph.

Some children who have sustained a head injury may also present signs suggestive of a chest injury. If abdominal distension is present, a film of the abdomen may show marked dilatation of the stomach. The gastric dilatation causes mechanical embarrassment of the breathing and rapid relief is produced by the insertion of a Ryle's tube. The amount of gas obtained is much smaller than the size of the stomach suggests but, if the abdomen is re-X-rayed after half-an-hour, the dilatation will no longer be present.

TREATMENT

The classification of chest injuries produced by Salpekar (*Table 7.1*) is of considerable help in establishing the severity of the injury and indicating the appropriate treatment. Essentially, he uses 4 grades of severity increasing from Grade I to Grade IV.

In Grade I, fractured ribs are not associated with any pulmonary damage and respiratory function is essentially normal. In Grade IV rib fractures are absent or small in number, but there is massive damage to the lungs and pleural cavity, associated with serious impairment of pulmonary function. This group has a high mortality rate. Grades II and III show increasing degrees of pulmonary damage and respiratory dysfunction with a corresponding increase in the degree of the complexity of treatment required.

When a patient with a major chest lesion has suffered major injuries of other systems, there will not be any response to the initial resuscitative measures until the chest injury has been brought under control. Blood gas analysis is helpful in assessing the progress of the chest injury, but if it is not available the patient must be treated using clinical judgement and X-rays as a guide.

Traumatic asphyxia (*Figure 7.4*) does not require any active treatment, provided the lungs and pleura are undamaged. The patient should be admitted for observation and any pulmonary complications dealt with as indicated below. The treatment of surgical emphysema is the treatment of the underlying chest pathology.

Grade I

Grade I injuries should be treated by analgesia. Admission should be considered in adults who sustain more than 6 fractured ribs, particularly if both sides are affected. In elderly patients 1 or 2 ribs are frequently broken above and below those visible on X-ray, and admission should be considered if more than 4 ribs are seen to be fractured on the X-rays. In all ages much depends on the patient's condition and response to the injury. The main risk to the patient is the development of pneumonic changes following local contusion, or collapse associated with diminished respiratory excursions because of pain. When breathing is extremely

Table 7.1

CLASSIFICATION OF CHEST TRAUMA (after SALPEKAR)

Grade	I	II	III	IV
Mechanical	Rib fractures	Multiple fracture ribs Pneumo- or haemothorax	'Stove-in-chest' 'Paradox' Pneumo- and haemothorax	Bilateral, often tension pneumo- and haemothorax Few rib fractures
Parenchymal	Unaffected	Segmental atelectasis Pulmonary oedema within 48–72 hours	Moderate degree of pulmonary contusion Pulmonary oedema within 24 hours	Bilateral, severe pulmonary contusion and intra-alveolar haemorrhage Pulmonary oedema within 6 hours
Blood gases	PaO_2 80–100 mmHg $PaCO_2$ 35–45 mmHg	70–80 mmHg 50 mmHg	60–80 mmHg 45–55 mmHg	30–40 mmHg LOW 50–60 mmHg HIGH
Respiratory state	Normal	CO_2 retention with mild hypoxia	Progressive CO_2 retention with hypoxia	Massive physiological 'shunt'

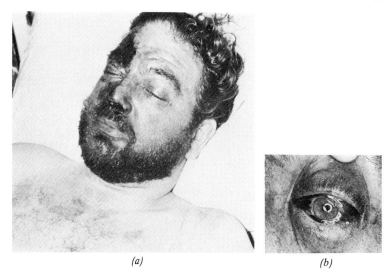

(a)   *(b)*

Figure 7.4.   *(a) Traumatic asphyxia. (b) Patient's eye, showing extensive conjunctival haemorrhages*

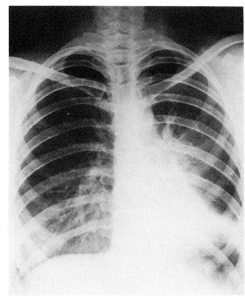

Figure 7.5. Small area of collapse of left lower lobe following localized contusion of the chest wall

painful and shallow, relief can be obtained by infiltrating the fracture areas with local anaesthetic. Alternatively, provided there is no pulmonary or pleural damage, a small dose (7.5–10.0 mg) of morphine should be given intravenously.

Every effort should be made to encourage the patient to remain physically active (though this may have to be at a reduced level) and deep breathing exercises are essential. Physiotherapy may be required if the patient is reluctant to move. Most of the patients in this grade can be treated as out-patients. Provided it is impressed on the patient that mobility and deep breathing are essential, the patients usually make a rapid recovery, but they must be warned that the pain may take rather longer to settle than they expect. Initial severe discomfort usually settles quickly, but complete freedom from pain may require 2 or 3 months.

Contusions of the chest, without visible rib damage on X-ray, requires similar management. The symptoms also take a surprisingly long time to disappear. From time to time a patient with fractured ribs may complain of coughing blood. This occurrence, at about 2 weeks after injury, arises from a small area of pulmonary contusion and is usually of little significance (*Figure 7.5*). Nevertheless, these patients should be followed up radiologically until the chest is clear.

Grade II

Grade II injuries require admission. Treatment is initially a matter of observation. A small pneumothorax or haemothorax does not require treatment in the Emergency Department but, when there is a large or tension pneumothorax present, a catheter, connected to an underwater seal, should be inserted into the pleural cavity (*Figure 7.6*). In an emergency, when a tension pneumothorax is present, a large-bore intravenous cannula should be inserted into the second intercostal space anteriorly, while arrangements are made to insert a self-retaining catheter and underwater seal into the same interspace. Alternatively, the catheter can be connected to a 'flutter' valve. This has the advantage that the patient can be ambulant, but it should not be used when blood is present otherwise the valve may become blocked by clots. Deep breathing exercises will help to expel the air in the pleural cavity. Alternatively, expansion of the lung can be assisted by the use of 10 cm of water negative pressure connected to the underwater seal.

It is unlikely that an isolated haemothorax will cause sufficient respiratory embarrassment to require drainage in the Emergency Department. They are usually part of Grades III and IV injury complexes, where the amount of blood lost may be sufficient to require replacement therapy. Their management is described later under these grades.

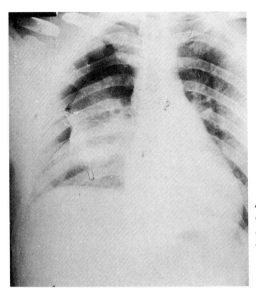

Figure 7.6. Grade II injury after drainage, showing pneumothorax and complete collapse of upper lobe on the right side

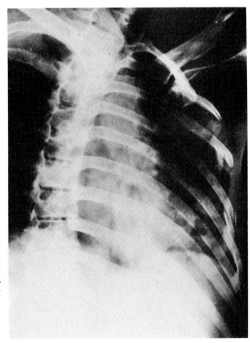

Figure 7.7. Grade III injury showing fractures of upper 5 ribs which were also fractured at the costochondral junction. Marked paradox was present

Grade III

Treatment should be commenced immediately it is clear that the patient falls into this group (*Figure 7.7*) A haemothorax of less than 500 ml is unlikely to show on the X-rays; therefore, if the X-ray shows a haemothorax, it is probable that the patient has lost at least 1 litre of blood into the thoracic cavity. The transfusion requirements should take into account haemorrhage from other injuries remembering the usual tendency to underestimate intrapleural blood loss.

A patient with a minor paradox affecting only 1 or 2 rib segments should be watched while blood gas estimations are carried out. If the PO_2 is 60 mmHg or above it is permissible to continue observation, but if the PO_2 is below this figure, or if the paradox is extensive, arrangements must be made for the patient to be mechanically ventilated. If the PO_2 is borderline, 50 per cent oxygen, given by a face mask, may produce sufficient improvement to avoid the necessity to ventilate the patient.

Ventilation

After the passage of a stomach tube and aspiration of the stomach contents, anaesthesia is induced with an intravenous anaesthetic. Intubation, using a cuffed endotracheal tube, is carried out under a short-acting muscle relaxant, after which the patient is connected to a ventilator. Long-acting muscle relaxants and intravenous sedatives are used to maintain the relaxation necessary for the ventilator to function. This procedure in an unprepared, seriously ill patient, frequently with blood-stained fluid in the upper air passages, is not one for the inexperienced junior doctor, and the services of a skilled anaesthetist should always be obtained when this injury requires treatment.

As soon as the patient is connected to the ventilator, the chest should be auscultated to ensure that the tube has not passed down the right main bronchus, leaving the left lung unventilated. If there is a complete absence of air entry on the left side, the tube should be withdrawn until sounds can be heard.

Pleural drainage

The increased inspiratory pressure caused by the ventilator may, if the lung is in any way damaged, force air into the pleural cavity, causing a tension pneumothorax. This condition can develop very quickly with mechanical ventilation, and it is essential that the affected pleural cavity or cavities are drained. Air can be released through a catheter, in each second interspace anteriorly, connected to an underwater seal. Unfortunately, in these cases the pleural cavity usually contains a significant amount of blood which will not drain through a catheter inserted high up anteriorly and another drain must be inserted lower down.

In an emergency, any type of self-retaining catheter can be used, and should be connected to an underwater seal. It is inserted in the sixth or seventh intercostal space behind the mid-axillary line.

Technique. Through an incision 2.5—4.0 cm long, parallel to the appropriate intercostal space, the tissues are divided down to the pleura. The catheter is then introduced into the pleural cavity in a manner appropriate to the cather being used. While an assistant connects it to the underwater seal, the operator sutures the skin around the catheter and either ties or tapes it to the chest wall to prevent it sliding in or out of the chest cavity. Ideally, a catheter specifically designed for intrapleural drainage should be used. These have an intrapleural length of about 10—15 cm, along which there are side holes. One or two inflatable cuffs may be fitted to provide a mechanical block to inwards or outwards sliding movements. This type of catheter is inserted in an upward direction in the sixth or seventh space and connected to the underwater seal. Air is evacuated through the tip of the catheter and blood drains through the side holes, thus avoiding the necessity to insert two catheters into the pleural cavity.

After treatment

Auscultation should be carried out at frequent intervals after the insertion of pleural drains. If drainage is proceeding satisfactory, the breath sounds will gradually re-appear and increase in strength.

Patchy areas or crepitation and bronchial breathing suggest patches of pulmonary contusion. X-Ray examination with the head end of the patient slightly raised should be carried out when the initial treatment is finished. Suction must be used to keep the air passages and endotracheal tube from becoming blocked by blood or other secretions, and blood replacement therapy should be continued at a rate dictated by the sum total of the injuries. Blood gas analysis should be used to check the response to the treatment. Humidification of the inspired air should be commenced as soon as possible to prevent inspissation of the secretions in the respiratory tract and the endotracheal tube.

It is usual, for a patient whose injury is in Grade III, to show marked improvement even in the presence of other major injuries, after treatment has been commenced. Failure to show such improvement raises other possibilities:

1. Has any other intrathoracic injury been overlooked, e.g. a rupture of the aorta or the diaphragm? On X-ray, the former shows broadening of the mediastinum; the latter may show abdominal contents in the pleural cavity.

2. Was the patient receiving any treatment prior to his accident from his practitioner or from another department in the hospital? If so, what was the disease and what were the drugs? For example, a patient with a coronary thrombosis might be receiving anticoagulant drugs. The patient might be a diabetic on insulin treatment or might be receiving steroids.

3. Did the patient have a coronary thrombosis before the accident? Has the patient sustained a cardiac contusion in the accident? The opinion of the medical unit might be required to help in excluding these conditions. Cardiac tamponade might be present if there is increasing venous distension and a falling blood pressure.

4. Is there an associated intra-abdominal lesion? This is a very difficult problem: the abdominal injury requires observation, the chest injury requires ventilation. Before intubation is carried out, the abdomen must be examined for evidence of injury. Rigidity must be noted and, if the patient is conscious, an attempt should be made to assess the possibility of an intra-abdominal lesion. When the lower left ribs are fractured posteriorly, the possibility of a ruptured spleen must be considered. If there is tenderness of the right upper abdomen, associated with rigidity, a ruptured liver may be suspected. Peritoneal lavage, which will not interfere with the treatment of the chest injury, can be carried out. A positive result will indicate that laparotomy is indicated; a negative result does not necessarily exclude an intra-abdominal lesion.

Once the patient's chest condition has been stabilized, the pulse rate should drop and the blood pressure should improve. If, after adequate blood replacement, these improvements do not occur, or if, after an initial improvement, they recurr, then the patient must be suffering from a progressive haemorrhage. Bleeding from chest and limb injuries can be seen; therefore the haemorrhage must be taking place in the abdominal cavity and laparotomy is indicated. If this is carried out through a small incision, a negative exploration will not affect the patient's recovery, whereas a failure to explore the abdomen could have serious consequences for the patient. Occasionally patients are lost by postponing laparotomy until the diagnosis is obvious. In the presence of a major chest injury, which requires immediate treatment, it is always safer to look and see and, if the junior doctor should consider that such a patient is being subjected to unnecessary delay, he should seek the assistance of his consultant, if he has not already done so. Considerable experience is necessary for the management of major chest lesions and, while a junior doctor might have to initiate treatment on his own responsibility, it is always preferable for him to obtain expert advice before he starts handling problems with which he is not familiar.

Grade IV

Patients with Grade IV injuries are seriously ill. They are dyspnoeic, cyanosed, restless and distressed. Frequently, a lilac colour is found on the side of the neck and ears. This colour which differs from cyanosis, is associated with severe pulmonary damage and disappears when mechanical ventilation is instituted. The physical signs in the chest are frequently bilateral. The breath sounds vary in intensity and patches of bronchial breathing, associated with râles, are commonly found.

Diminution of the breath sounds is found in collapse, haemothorax and haemopneumothorax. High-pitched sounds suggest a tension pneumothorax. Paradoxical respiration is not present, but areas of contusion may be found on the chest wall. Blood gas analysis shows a very low PO_2 level – figures of around 40 mmHg being common. The PCO_2 may show a slight rise to 50 mmHg; a high level at this stage always suggests the possibility, in elderly persons, of pre-existing pulmonary disease. X-Ray examination may or may not be helpful at this stage (*Figure 7.8*). Spectacular rib injuries are not present but 2 or 3 ribs may be fractured, frequently associated with surgical emphysema. The absence of rib fractures does not exclude severe pulmonary damage. If a reasonable film is obtained, this will show a patchy mottling of the lung fields (*Figure 7.9*). This may occupy the major part of both lungs but it is important to realize that this mottling indicates pulmonary damage due to contusion of the lungs. Segmental atelectasis and intra-alveolar haemorrhage occur which, when associated with pulmonary shunts, seriously interfere with both blood oxygenation and carbon dioxide excretion; X-rays, taken at intervals, will show a marked increase in the degree of mottling. If the initial changes seem to be minor in nature, but occupy the majority of the lung fields, the doctor can be sure that within 12 hours the changes will be extensive and little normal lung tissue will be visible.

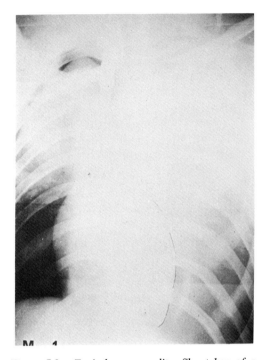

Figure 7.8. Typical poor quality film taken of a patient with a severe chest injury. This shows right apical pneumothorax and a complete opacity of the left side of the chest. After a large tension haemopneumothorax was treated on the left side, it could be seen that the left lung was completely collapsed. Drainage of the right pleural cavity demonstrated a similar, though less severe condition, which was associated with complete collapse of the upper lobe. This patient had profound pulmonary oedema and ventilation and pleural drainage were initiated immediately he arrived in the department. In severe chest injuries, even poor quality portable films may be of assistance in the initial management

A haemothorax will obscure the underlying lung tissues; an estimate of the size of the haemorrhage is not possible on emergency films, but when present on both sides indicates that both sides of the chest require drainage.

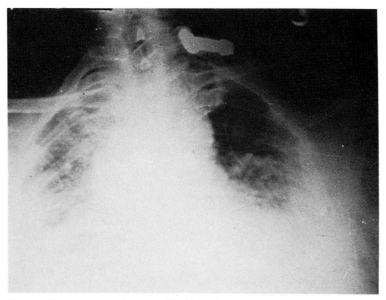

Figure 7.9.   A poor quality portable film taken with the patient lying flat. This showed marked contusion of the right lung and similar, though less marked, changes in the lower lobe of the left lung

Treatment

Treatment must be commenced as soon as possible. If the patient's condition is serious, and particularly when it is associated with other major injuries, it must be based on clinical assessment. Intravenous therapy should be commenced using a plasma substitute until blood is available. If more than 4 pints of blood are needed, the blood should be warmed and filtered.

The cyanosis cannot be removed by oxygen given through a face mask. In contrast to Grade III, where the problem is primarily mechanical affecting the rib cage with limited pulmonary damage, patients in Grade IV have minimal mechanical disability, but gross disturbance in the gaseous diffusion functions of the lungs, caused by segmental collapse, intra-alveolar haemorrhage, and the presence of blood and other secretions in the bronchial tract. The PO_2 can only be raised by the institution of mechanical ventilation through an endotracheal tube using a high level of humidified oxygen. A very high inflation pressure may be necessary to produce adequate inflation; skill is required to insert the tube and adjust the ventilator. It is inadvisable for the junior doctor to attempt to manage such a patient and the assistance of a skilled anaesthetist should always be obtained.

As soon as the patient is on the ventilator, one or both sides of the pleural cavity should be drained as described for Group III cases. The blood gas estimations should be repeated after 1 hour, and an attempt should be made to obtain good quality X-ray films of the chest as soon as the initial stages of management are over. If the patient's chest is raised slightly, films can be produced on a mobile X-ray machine which will give some indication of the degree of lung damage and of the state of the pleural cavity.

The positive pressure ventilation will, by inflating the lungs, drive out the air and/or blood from the pleural cavity. If the patient's condition is improving, it is probable that the PO_2 will have risen to between 50 and 60 mmHg and the lung fields will be clearer though mottling and a haemothorax may still be present. If the PO_2 has not changed, it is unlikely that there will be any significant change in the X-rays. The haemothorax may be less, but the changes of pulmonary contusion will be more marked and occupy a greater area of the lung fields. The PO_2 may also show an increase and changes indicative of a respiratory and metabolic acidosis may also develop. The prognosis for a patient exhibiting these changes is grave, since they indicate that pulmonary gas diffusion is markedly impaired and is not responding to treatment.

Tracheal toilet is essential from the beginning. Blood and secretions will easily block the endotracheal tube and, in order to avoid the secretions drying out, humidification of the inspired gases should be commenced at an early stage. The risk of infection is high; therefore sterile disposable plastic gloves and a fresh soft catheter should be used each time bronchial toilet is carried out. Damage to the bronchial lining is avoided by inserting the catheter to its full depth and then gently withdrawing it. The tube should not be pushed in and out repetitively; this causes unnecessary damage to the bronchial epithelium and can increase the bleeding.

The Emergency Department must be prepared to deal with such a patient until the initial treatment has been carried out on the respiratory injury. Other major injuries cannot be dealt with until the patient's condition improves and this will not occur until the blood oxygenation approaches 60 mmHg. A PO_2 of near 40 mmHg is approaching the level which will not support life and the longer the PO_2 is allowed to remain at a low level, the greater the damage that will be caused by hypoxia. Oxygen diffusion across tissues depends on the partial pressure of the gas in the blood: when tissues are damaged and the partial pressure is extremely low, hypoxic damage will be caused in many tissues which produces complex problems of a biochemical and a haematological nature during the patient's subsequent treatment. It is therefore important that the initial care of the patient should display an awareness of the problem that extends beyond the immediate confines of the Emergency Department.

8

Abdominal and Pelvic Trauma

Injuries to the abdomen neatly divide themselves into 'open' and 'closed'. Every open wound and closed contusion is significant enough to justify physical examination.

Open injuries

It is rare for a patient to arrive with a prolapsed bowel, and a recent penetrating injury or stab wound of the abdomen may look quite innocent on the surface (*Figure 8.1*). What matters is not the *length* of the skin wound but its *depth*. All wounds must be explored to ascertain

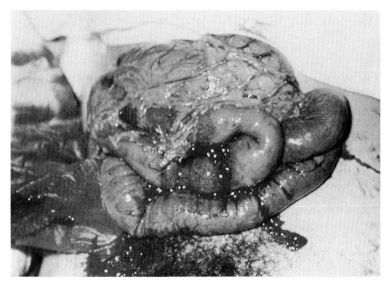

Figure 8.1. Stab wound of abdomen with prolapse of intestines. Despite the spectacular nature of the wound, minimal damage was caused to the intestines and the patient made a rapid recovery

whether or not they have entered the peritoneal cavity and, if they have, a formal laparotomy is required. A small wound of the bowel will produce very few symptoms until peritonitis develops several hours later, by which time the patient may have left hospital if the implications of the skin wound were not appreciated. These remarks apply particularly to gun shot wounds. Remember the simple mathematical calculation that the number of entry-wounds minus the number of exit-wounds equals the number of bullets still in the body. A radiological examination in the erect position will not only show metallic foreign bodies but may also reveal free gas under the diaphragm if the bowel has been damaged.

Closed injuries

Any patient who complains of abdominal pain after a blow on the abdomen, especially if he vomits, must be examined and observed as a potential case of 'ruptured viscus'. The condition is most common in young men but can occur at any age. Road traffic accidents, works accidents, sport or play accidents, falls and assaults are the main causes, listed in descending order of frequency.

HISTORY

If the patient can recall and describe the injury this may give a lead as to the possible damage. A steering wheel blow into the upper abdomen may rupture the liver or spleen or crush the small bowel or pancreas against the vertebral column. The length of time since the injury occurred is also important: it may take up to 4 hours for the symptoms to become definite. After this time the only remaining risk of undeclared symptoms is from 'delayed rupture of the spleen' which is described later.

PHYSICAL EXAMINATION

This begins with *inspection*. Remember to assess the whole patient, looking particularly for evidence of trauma to the head and thorax as well as the abdomen. Pulse, blood pressure and especially respiration should be examined and recorded with a note of the time at which the observations were made. The shocked patient with suspected internal blood loss demands a blood transfusion. A good intravenous line should be established in the upper limb before attempting to decide whether the bleeding is into the thorax or abdomen or both. Marks on the skin of the chest or abdomen from the imprint of clothing are very significant — they imply severe trauma and visceral damage is extremely likely; but their absence is of no significance. The presence of bruising should be noted.

Palpation

This will elicit localized tenderness and should include 'springing' the pelvis and palpating the pubic rami. Blood loss from a fractured pelvis is often of the order of a litre or more and this injury is frequently associated with other abdominal trauma, especially rupture of the diaphragm when excessive force has produced a 'blow-out' of the abdomen. While palpating the abdomen, enquiry should be made about radiation of the pain and specific questions should be asked about pain felt behind the shoulders. Bruising or tearing of the diaphragm or damage to the liver or spleen frequently produce referred pain to the back of the respective shoulders.

Percussion

If testing for 'shifting dullness' indicates that there is free fluid in the abdomen following trauma, one can assume that the fluid in question is blood. With the patient lying supine, a ball-point pen is used to make a mark on the skin where the percussion note changes from resonant to dull as the percussing fingers pass from the umbilicus to the loin. The patient is then turned on his side and after a minute the examination is repeated, this time percussing from the upper loin towards the umbilicus and beyond. Again the point of change from resonant to dull is noted. A distance of more than 5 cm between the first and second marks is significant.

Auscultation

Probably the most important single physical finding following trauma to the abdomen is absence of the bowel sounds. No conclusions can be drawn if they are heard, but if, after listening carefully for 2—3 minutes, no sounds are heard the patient must at least remain under observation. Most significant of all, if the bowel sounds were initially present but subsequently disappear, visceral damage is present.

INVESTIGATIONS

Radiological examination will show loss of the psoas shadows on the supine film if there is a large haemoperitoneum. Fractures of the pelvis or the lower ribs, which encase the liver and spleen, will be demonstrated. The erect film will show air under the diaphragm if the gut is torn or, 2–3 hours after the injury, fluid levels in the bowel will be seen if damage to the mesentry has devitalized a portion of the gut. A serum amylase of over 1.000 Somogyi units implies damage to the pancreas and such an injury is often accompanied by damage to the overlying mesentry and small bowel.

Haematological examinations, other than grouping and cross-matching blood, are not particularly helpful in the acute stage. Haemoglobin and haematocrit levels can be useful as baseline information, but the rate and quantity of blood replacement is better monitored by the patient's clinical response and the readings from a central venous catheter.

Peritoneal lavage is now gaining wide acceptance and has largely replaced the four quadrant tap as a direct method of establishing the presence of a haemoperitoneum, but it should not be used during pregnancy or when there has been a previous mid-line laparotomy. The technique for performing peritoneal lavage is:

1. Catheterize the bladder.
2. Infiltrate local anaesthetic into the skin and subcutaneous tissues down to the peritoneum at a point 5 cm below the umbilicus.
3. Make a stab incision down to the peritoneum.
4. Introduce a peritoneal dialysis trochar and cannula into the wound and through the peritoneum, aiming in a caudal direction, towards the pelvis.
5. Having penetrated the peritoneum, withdraw the tip of the trochar and advance the cannula, with the trochar still inside it, until all the irrigation holes are within the peritoneal cavity. Then withdraw the trochar completely.
6. Connect a half litre plastic sac of warm saline to the cannula and run it in as quickly as it will go. Tip the patient slightly head-down for about 1 minute.
7. Just before the last of the saline runs into the abdomen, take the plastic sac off the drip stand and place it on the floor.
8. Observe the colour of the fluid which syphons out. If there is a haemoperitoneum it will return bright red.
9. Apart from observing the evidence of a haemoperitoneum, the return fluid can be studied for the presence of cells, amylase or bile.

Examination of the urine should not be overlooked. Macroscopic haematuria is diagnostic evidence of renal injury if there is pain and tenderness in the loin.

Throughout the period of investigation and observation 5 basic measurements should be repeated at half-hour intervals:

Pulse.
Blood pressure.
Respiration.
Abdominal girth.
Abdominal auscultation for bowel sounds.

In the severe case the need for laparotomy will have quickly become evident but in the less severe case these repeated observations, after 3—4 hours, will have established one of three patterns:

1. There has been a slow steady deterioration — laparotomy is indicated.
2. The observations, although not normal, have remained at a steady level — admission to a surgical ward for continued observation over a 24-hour period must be arranged.
3. The observations have remained or returned to normal. Preparations can be made for the patient to go home.

ABDOMINAL INJURY AS ONE OF MULTIPLE INJURIES

From what has been written it must now be obvious that if there are other dramatic injuries, such as a dislocated hip or an open fracture of the leg, there is a risk that the patient may already be under a general anaesthetic for the treatment of these peripheral injuries before the presence of an intra-abdominal lesion can be fully appreciated. Yet it is the slowly developing visceral lesion which may kill the patient rather than the bone sticking out through the trouser leg. All surgeons treating injured patients must be aware of the risk of central trauma being overlooked because of the more obvious peripheral injuries, and above all they must be cognisant of the responsibility they take when arranging for a general anaesthetic to be given to a patient who has been recently injured. An anaesthetized patient cannot complain of increasing abdominal pain and all the vital signs will be confused by the surgical act and the anaesthetic.

DELAYED RUPTURE OF THE SPLEEN

One unsolved problem in the management of abdominal injury patients is what to do about 'delayed rupture of the spleen'. If a patient sustains a blow over the spleen, there is a small localized splenic haemorrhage; the splenic area is tender but the vital signs are unaffected. After a period of observation the tenderness begins to subside and the patient goes home. Days or even weeks later (5 weeks later in one patient in our experience) the spleen tears open, the peritoneal cavity fills with blood and urgent transfusion and splenectomy are required to save the patient's life. Radiology may be helpful in attempting to predict this possible late development. A tethered left diaphragm or an enlarged splenic shadow following trauma to the upper abdomen should either result in an exploratory laparotomy or else advice should be given to the patient not to travel far from skilled surgical care in the subsequent 2 months.

TRAUMA TO THE URINARY TRACT

Macroscopic haematuria in a patient who is tender over the kidney following trauma is to be regarded as diagnostic proof of a ruptured kidney. All such patients should be admitted to hospital; nearly all of them can be managed conservatively. An intravenous pyelogram will demonstrate the degree and severity of the damage. Occasionally, if the haematuria is massive or persists for many days, renal surgery will become necessary.

The ureters are well protected from blunt trauma but rarely a stone lurking in the renal pelvis is dislodged during a traumatic episode and enters the ureter producing the classical picture of renal colic. The management and treatment is the same as for other patients with ureteric calculus.

RUPTURE OF THE BLADDER

Intraperitoneal rupture is usually a late night injury. Someone who has drunk too much alcohol has an overfull bladder and staggers in front of a motor vehicle. The distended bladder bursts emptying urine into the abdominal cavity. The patient arrives at hospital with severe lower abdominal pain and may well be shocked.

Extraperitoneal rupture is more common and is a complication of fracture of the pelvis. This injury of itself is less shocking to the patient but he has an urgent desire to urinate. Despite repeated efforts no urine is produced, but a drop of blood may emerge at the external meatus. Gradually it becomes obvious that urine is being extravasated into surrounding tissues. Both forms of rupture can be confirmed by retrograde cystoscopy and they require urgent surgical repair.

RUPTURE OF THE URETHRA

This is also mentioned in Chapter 14 when discussing fractures of the pelvis, but urethral rupture may also be caused by falling astride a hard object. Pain, bruising and swelling in the perineum and a drop of blood appearing at the external meatus suggest the diagnosis which can be confirmed by radiological urethrography. Recent opinion is that suprapubic catheterization is preferable to attempting to pass a urethral catheter as the latter may compound the injury and also introduce infection.

9

Injuries to the Back and Neck

Patients come to the Accident and Emergency Department with disorders of the back and neck for one of two reasons:

1. They have been involved in a violent accident.
or 2. They have had a sudden spontaneous onset of pain.

In either group there may be few physical signs and, of course, in the unconscious patient there are no symptoms. This means that the doctor who manages these patients must have a clear understanding of the nature of the conditions and a definitie routine to follow.

SPINAL INJURIES

These follow violent accidents and include one or more of the following elements:

1. A fracture of the bones of the spine.
2. Tearing of the ligaments which give stability to the spine.
3. Damage to the spinal cord.

Causes

Falls from a height — such as from a roof, a ladder, scaffolding, a tree or head forwards downstairs.

Objects falling onto a patient — such as bags of cement or corn, packing cases or drums falling onto the shoulders when the spine is flexed.

Road traffic accidents — although traffic accidents often produce multiple injuries, the patient may have been thrown out of the car or off a motorcycle and have suffered only an acute flexion injury of the spine.

Whiplash injury of the neck — when a patient is sitting in a stationary vehicle which is hit from behind by another vehicle travelling at speed, the impact causes the neck to be jerked backwards into hyperextension, straining or tearing the anterior longitudinal ligament which may result in a subluxation. These patients often walk into hospital complaining of pain in the neck when no other injury is present.

Sports injuries — particularly the contact sports such as rugby but also diving may cause injury to the spine.

Routine of management of a patient with a suspected spinal injury

Any patient who gives a history of an accident similar to those listed above and who complains of pain in the neck or back, and particularly if he complains of numbness or tingling in the arms or legs, should be managed in the following way:

1. If the patient has not been brought in on a trolley, he must be helped onto one and required to lie down immediately, even if he considers that one is making an unnecessary fuss.
2. Adequate 'man-power' should be available (doctors, nurses, porters, students, ambulance men) so that the patient can be eased up gently from the trolley as the clothes are being removed. The patient must not be allowed to sit up.
3. While this man-power is available a carrying sheet should be inserted under the patient if this has not already been done. The patient is turned very gently onto one side and the rolled-up carrying sheet is placed over half the trolley. While the patient is in this position, the spine and posterior ribs are palpated for points of tenderness. The patient is then rolled gently onto the other side so that the carrying sheet can be unrolled to cover the rest of the trolley. Carrying poles are now inserted so that the patient can be lifted onto the X-ray table and into bed without risking further damage to the spine.
4. If a lesion of the cervical spine is suspected, a reliable assistant should stand at the head of the trolley and exert gentle traction on the neck with one hand under the chin and the other hand under the occiput. After all movements for undressing and examination of the patient have been completed, the head is wedged between sandbags.

Further clinical examination

For spinal cord damage.   Reflexes and movements should be checked in both upper and lower limbs to detect signs of paralysis. Fractures of the long bones may prevent a complete test of movements, but movements of wrist and fingers, ankles and toes can nearly always be achieved even in the presence of fractures. If any sign of paralysis is discovered, cutaneous sensation to pin prick should be tested, and areas of anaesthesia noted.

For further injuries.   If the patient has multiple injuries, the routine as described in Chapter 2 should be carried out.

X-Ray examination

In the resuscitation room, X-ray examination is greatly facilitated by the use of fluoroscopy and an image intensifier to scan the spine. If such equipment is not available, then the whole spine must be X-rayed and films developed. Remember that there may be injuries at two different levels and the radiological examination must not be abandoned when the first lesion is found. It is often difficult to obtain a lateral view of the seventh cervical and first thoracic vertebrae because they are obscured by the shoulders. The radiographer may require assistance to pull down on the arms and lower the shoulders so that these vertebrae can be clearly seen in this view.

Scrutiny of X-ray films

Cervical region

1. On the lateral view, examine the anterior border of the body of each vertebra for any sign of wedging or collapse or detachment of a small piece of bone. The 'tear drop' fracture from one corner of the anterior border of a vertebral body usually signifies that there has also been an avulsion of the anterior longitudinal ligament and rupture of the intervertebral disc. Such a lesion means that the spine is quite unstable and special care must be taken to keep the cervical spine at rest until the patient is firmly fixed in bed. Degenerative changes in the discs, with loss of disc space and osteophytic outgrowths, can be noted and serve as a guide to later treatment.
2. Now examine the alignment of the posterior borders of the vertebrae. Normally this line makes a gentle continuous curve.

An abrupt change at one level in this curved line or a step from one vertebra to the next, is evidence of a subluxation. Remember that the bones do not need to be fractured for there to be a potentially disastrous, unstable lesion if the ligaments are torn (*Figure 9.1*). Minor degrees of instability will be demonstrated by flexion and extension films taken under medical supervision when the original X-rays do not show any abnormality.

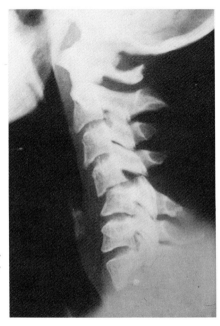

Figure 9.1. Dislocation of the cervical spine without any bony injury

3. The neural arch of each vertebra and the intervertebral joints should be examined next. If there is any doubt in the interpretation of the films, oblique views will be helpful. Finally, on this view, look for the rare occurrence of a fractured spinous process.
4. The antero-posterior (A-P) view should show a regular symmetrical alignment of the vertebrae. An A-P view through the mouth must always be included to show the odontoid process and the atlanto-axial joints. Special scrutiny of the base of the odontoid process should be made for signs of fracture, the relationship of the atlanto-axial joints to the odontoid process must be symmetrical, and the relationship of this process to the arch of the atlas must be checked on the lateral view.

Thoracic and lumbar regions

1. On the lateral view, search for a wedge-shaped collapse of a vertebral body. Old people, or those on long-term steroid therapy, may already have one or more collapsed vertebrae due to osteoporosis, so it is important to correlate the radiological appearance with the physical signs. If a suspicious wedge-shaped vertebra is found at the upper or lower border of the X-ray film, another view should be taken with the suspected vertebra in the centre of the film.

2. Examine the laminae and spinous processes for evidence of fracture.

3. The A-P view may reveal the collapse of a vertebral body. More often there is a scoliosis of the spine centred at the point of fracture. If such a scoliosis exists, the lateral view must be scrutinized again to ensure no fracture at this point has been missed.

4. In the lumbar region each transverse process of the vertebra should be inspected in turn for fracture.

5. Finally, any ribs visible on the X-rays should be examined individually for signs of fracture.

Initial treatment of spinal injuries

Fractures of vertebral bodies and subluxation

Without paraplegia.   The management of these patients depends not so much on the bony injury itself but on whether or not the spinal cord is at risk. The patient who has suffered the partial collapse of one vertebral body should be told that the injury is minimal. Such a patient will only require bed rest for 7 to 10 days followed by a similar period of physiotherapy. In consultation with the orthopaedic surgeon a decision may even be taken to manage the patient at home and so avoid admission to hospital. Conversely, the patient with a potentially unstable fracture or even a slight degree of subluxation following a ligamentous injury requires the utmost care and attention from the A & E Department doctor. Responsibility for such a patient includes supervising his transport to the ward and handing him over personally to the orthopaedic surgeon or to a senior member of the nursing staff on the ward.

With paraplegia.   Patients who have substained damage to the spinal cord, irrespective of the X-ray appearance, are best admitted without delay to the Spinal Injuries Unit if this can be arranged. Only if the transfer of the patient will be delayed for several hours should the bladder be catheterized, and this procedure should be done under full aseptic conditions after telephone consultation with the staff of the Spinal Injuries Unit. During this initial period before transfer, the patient must be turned at 2 hourly intervals to avoid developing pressure sores.

Fractures of the transverse processes of lumbar vertebrae

It is important that the term 'fractured spine' should never be used for these patients. In all of them the urine should be examined for macroscopic haematuria to find out if the injury has also produced a rupture of the kidney. In the absence of this complication the patient can be told that he has bruised his back or that a very small piece of bone has been pulled away from the spine. He will need bed rest and possibly analgesic tablets for a week followed by a week or two or rehabilitation, and should be able to return to heavy work within a month. It will be much longer if the patient thinks he has a fractured spine or has 'broken his back'.

Clay shoveller's fracture

This is a fracture of the spinous process of the seventh cervical or first dorsal vertebrae found in men like clay shovellers who are heaving heavy loads with their arms. Acute tenderness is found over the process and an X-ray shows the detached bony fragment. Treatment is by an injection of local anaesthetic and a soft collar until pain and tenderness disappear.

SPONTANEOUS PAIN IN THE NECK AND BACK

Patients with acute pain in the neck or back attend Accident and Emergency Departments every day. To avoid missing the few patients who have a serious condition, it is necessary to examine them all. It will speed up the process if those with cervical or thoracic pain are stripped to the waist before the doctor sees them, and those with lumbar pain are undressed as far as their underclothes and lying on a trolley.

Acute wry neck or torticollis

This well known condition often occurs as a patient is getting out of bed or dressing in the morning. It occurs at all ages and in both sexes. The head is held with the chin pointing to one shoulder. Attempts to twist the head to the opposite side cause acute pain and spasm in the neck. Physical examination should first exclude an underlying ear or throat infection. Then the muscle spasm can be relieved by using a cold 'pain relieving' spray applied over the neck muscles on the side away from the chin until the first sign of frostiness appears. As the neck warms again, the patient is instructed to move it freely. If there is slight residual stiffness, manipulation of the neck with the patient lying down and traction applied by one hand under the chin and the other under the occiput, usually completes the cure. A soft collar may be worn for 2 to 3 days if the neck is still uncomfortable.

Cervical spondylosis

Degenerative changes in the cervical spine are increasingly common beyond the age of 45 to 50 years. The condition may have been symptomless until it is brought to light by a trivial blow or twisting injury, or a road traffic accident. In other patients the pain develops spontaneously. If there is pressure on the cervical nerve roots there may be pain referred to the arms, the shoulder region or between the shoulder blades. Often the patient only complains of the referred pain and is suprised by the suggestion that the root of the trouble is in the neck.

Physical examination must include noting down the range of movement in the neck in the 6 directions of: flexion, extension, rotation to right and left, and lateral flexion to both sides. If pain is referred to the arm, reflexes, muscle power and joint movement should be examined and compared with the opposite arm and the findings recorded. X-Ray examination will very probably show the degenerative changes in the cervical spine, but the radiological appearance often bears little relation to the severity of the symptoms.

Treatment

In consultation with orthopaedic colleagues, the A & E Department staff may undertake the early treatment of these patients. The principles of treatment are rest, pain relief and measures to improve the circulation and thereby probably to reduce the oedema around the nerve roots. Rest for the neck is provided by applying a cervical collar which is adjusted to hold the head in the most comfortable position. It is important for the patient to be able to sleep, and if he is more comfortable in the collar he should wear it through the night; analgesic tablets should also be prescribed to ensure sleep. By the end of the second week the patient should start to wean himself of the collar by wearing it a little less on each successive day. If symptoms persist, physiotherapy is indicated. Traction and/or manipulation of the neck help some patients but seem to exacerbate the symptoms in others. Diapulse therapy is proving to be a valuable means of easing the pain in the neck, presumably by dispersing the oedema around the nerve roots.

Low back pain

This common complaint is usually provoked by lifting with the back flexed. It may be due to a muscle strain, to oedema or to haematoma or, occasionally, to a prolapsed intervertebral disc.

Physical examination

While the patient is lying down, test for reduction in straight leg raising; only if the range is less than 60° is it of real significance. Examine the knee, ankle and plantar reflexes. Test for weakness in extension or flexion of the big toes, and for diminished sensation in the legs or feet. Because the pain may be partially related to the hip joint, test the range of movement in both hips. If the patient can stand, look for scoliosis, kyphosis and the loss of the normal lumbar lordosis. Palpate the spine for local tenderness and test the movements of spinal flexion, extension, lateral flexion to left and right, and rotation.

X-Ray examination

This should be done more to exclude bony abnormality, disease or secondary deposits than for any direct help in diagnosis because, as in the neck, degenerative changes often bear little relation to the severity of the symptoms.

Treatment

In low back pain the sheet anchor of treatment is rest in bed on a firm mattress. This can usually be arranged at home. Occasionally, for the patient with a prolapsed intervertebral disc, an orthopaedic surgeon may prefer to admit the patient to hospital for bed rest, traction, analgesia and further assessment with a view to laminectomy. In the rare cases of a central disc prolapse producing urinary retention, urgent operative treatment will be necessary, but by far the majority of patients will be treated by conservative methods. Following a period of bed rest, rehabilitation in the Physiotherapy Department will speed up recovery. Supervised exercises in a pool heated to 35°C is probably the most beneficial single form of treatment. Traction, manipulation, graded exercises and electrotherapy may all have a part to play. Finally, weight reduction and regular physical exercise, particularly swimming, are to be recommended to diminish the risk of recurrent attacks of low back pain.

10

Injuries to the Shoulder

Pain around the shoulder may result from an accident or from localized degenerative changes which are often brought to light by small repeated injuries or by abnormal use, such as painting a ceiling.

The symptoms can be conveniently classified as arising principally from:

1. The bones.
2. The joints.
3. The soft tissues.

Fractures or dislocations will be confirmed by X-ray examination but it must be remembered that:

1. Following an accident there may be more important injuries elsewhere — such as, for instance, a ruptured spleen.
2. Serious soft tissue injuries around the shoulder may be associated with the abnormality shown on the X-ray, particularly damage to nerves.
3. A 'negative' X-ray does not mean that 'there is nothing wrong'. Soft tissue lesions causing pain and disability still require examination, diagnosis and treatment.

HISTORY

The time elapsed since the injury

If more than 24 hours have passed since the injury, the possibility of other serious lesions being present without symptoms is remote. Patients with dislocations and some fractures around the shoulder joint may not come for treatment until several days after the accident. In some of the localized degenerative changes the pain comes on suddenly without any specific injury, in others the symptoms develop gradually over several weeks.

The type of accident

In road traffic accidents, or other accidents producing generalized bodily trauma, the pain in the shoulder may mask symptoms of other serious lesions. Head injuries, damage to viscera and the spine may occasionally produce few symptoms in recent accidents of this type. When the possibility of their presence is remembered, further questioning and examination will lead to their discovery.

When the accident is confined to the shoulder itself, there may be local complications. A violent traction injury may result in lesions of the brachial plexus. Wrenching of the shoulder causing increasing pain suggests a rotator cuff injury. A violent muscular effort in which the patient feels something 'give', suggests a tendon rupture.

PHYSICAL EXAMINATION

Satisfactory examination of the shoulder requires removal of all clothes from the upper part of the trunk. The routine for the removal of the clothes is to take them off the sound side, which is able to be moved without pain. Then bring the clothes over the head and finally slide them down the painful limb. (In redressing, the painful side is clothed first.)

As in the examination of any joint, there are 4 successive stages — look, feel, move, X-ray — which are considered in detail below.

Look

Deformity, swelling, bruising or scars should be detected and recorded.

Deformity of the arm with abduction at the shoulder suggests a dislocation or fracture of the neck of the humerus. An angular contour to the shoulder, replacing the normal rounded shape, is further evidence of a dislocated shoulder (*Figure 10.1*). Occasionally, careful observation may suggest that the dislocation is posterior rather than anterior (*Figure 10.2*).

Deformity of the clavicle at the site of fracture with downward sagging of the shoulder is often obvious in fracture of the middle third of the clavicle. Acromio-clavicular dislocation produces an obvious lump: the outer end of the clavicle is raised compared with the opposite side. Similarly, sterno-clavicular dislocation produces an asymmetry of the two adjacent sterno-clavicular joints.

Swelling around the shoulder joint is seen when there is a fracture of the neck of the humerus: the normal curvature of the shoulder, when seen from behind, is fuller or more rounded. A more localized swelling over the front of the point of the shoulder is caused by fluid in the sub-acromial bursa.

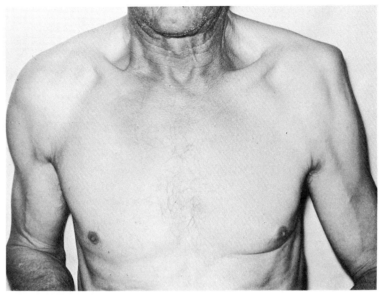

Figure 10.1.   Dislocation of the left shoulder

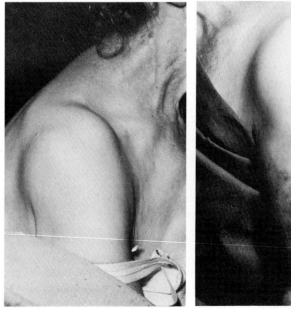

Figure 10.2   *Figure 10.3*

Bruising is rarely seen in very recent injuries. It usually takes 2 to 3 days to develop and is then useful in diagnosis. *Figure 10.3* shows a patient in whom bleeding has taken place deep to the deltoid muscle. The blood has tracked down the arm to come to the surface below the deltoid insertion. If X-ray fails to reveal a fracture, then this bleeding has come from a rupture of tendon or muscle deep to the deltoid, that is from the rotator cuff muscles or the long head of biceps.

Feel

Obvious swellings are palpated first to discover associated tenderness. When flattening of the curve of the shoulder suggests dislocation, palpation of the sub-coracoid region or the axilla may reveal the head of the humerus lying outside the joint and the examining fingers can be pressed in under the arch of the acromion.

When no obvious deformities or swellings are present, the bones should be palpated in turn to discover points of tenderness. Acute local tenderness on the subcutaneous border of the clavicle following a recent injury is evidence of a fracture or sub-periosteal haematoma. Even if the injury does not show on X-ray the patient requires a triangular sling to rest the arm until the pain settles. Occasionally, a greenstick fracture in a child can only be detected on X-ray when callus forms 10 days later. All points of tenderness should be recorded as guides to subsequent treatment.

Fracture of the neck of the humerus, or more usually dislocation of the shoulder joint, may be complicated by damage to the circumflex humeral nerve. This results in an area of anaesthesia over the upper outer aspect of the arm overlying the deltoid muscle and partial paralysis of this muscle. It is important to test for the presence of this complication before performing any manipulation lest the patient subsequently attributes the anaesthesia and weakness to the manipulation rather than the accident. The pattern of anaesthesia and paralysis in the rest of the upper limb will give diagnostic detail when there is a lesion of the brachial plexus.

Move

Following recent trauma, movements of the shoulder joint may be impossible or extremely painful and of little or no diagnostic value. *Figure*

Figure 10.2. Posterior dislocation of the shoulder. Note the hollow anteriorly, and the prominence of the head of the humerus posteriorly

Figure 10.3. Bruising from a shoulder injury. The blood has tracked down deep to the deltoid muscle before reaching the surface

10.4 shows the characteristic way in which a patient supports the dislocated arm, with the opposite hand under the elbow, so as to reduce the pain. Conversely, for the patient with pain arising from a localized degenerative lesion, testing and recording the range of movement is the most important part of the examination. It is essential, therefore, that it is done correctly in a standardized manner, and recorded systematically.

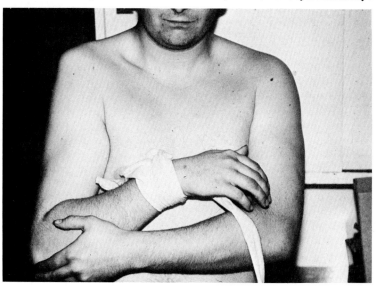

Figure 10.4.   Dislocation of the right shoulder. The patient is supporting the arm with the opposite hand under the elbow, to reduce the pain of the dislocation

This part of the examination will establish the diagnosis and form a baseline for assessing the patient's progress. The internationally accepted convention for examining and recording joint movement is described in the booklet *Joint Motion, Method of Measuring and Recording,* published by the American Academy of Orthopaedic Surgeons, Churchill Livingstone, 1976.

To examine movements of the shoulder joint, stand behind the patient and perform the movements of flexion and abduction with him. If abduction is limited, fix the scapula to the chest wall to determine whether the movement is taking place at the scapulo-thoracic or the scapulo-humeral joints. Internal and external rotation are most accurately examined with the shoulder abducted to a right-angle and the eblow flexed to 90° (*Figure 10.5*). Now record the range of active and passive movement and note which movements, or parts of a movement, are painful.

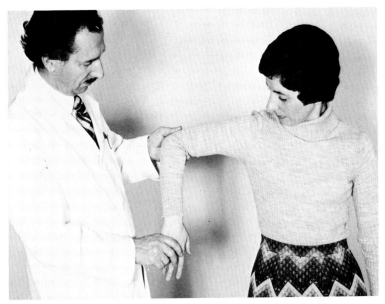

Figure 10.5.   Examination of internal rotation of the shoulder

In the presence of a brachial plexus lesion, movement in the rest of the upper limb must be examined and recorded.

X-Ray examination

For most radiological examinations of the shoulder one antero-posterior exposure is sufficient, but to this can be added an 'axial view' with the X-ray source above the shoulder and the film in the axilla. Unfortunately, the patient with a dislocated shoulder cannot abduct his arm to permit an axial view so a 'trans-thoracic view' is used. For this the uninjured arm is held above the head and the film cassette positioned on the outer aspect of the injured shoulder. This view is particularly important in diagnosing a posterior dislocation of the shoulder.

TREATMENT

This will be discussed in three sections:

1. Lesions of the bones, i.e. fractures.
2. Lesions of the joints.
3. Lesions of the soft tissues.

Fractures

Fracture of the clavicle — a broken collar bone — is one of the commonest fractures of childhood. It has been customary to treat this fracture by applying 'a figure-of-eight' bandage to brace back the shoulders and thereby pull the clavicle out to length. This treatment is effective but very uncomfortable. We have found in recent years that simply supporting the arm in a triangular sling is sufficient. Once the weight of the arm is taken from the shoulder and supported by the sling, the muscles attached to the clavicle pull the bony fragments into line, and in a child, the fracture heals in 3 weeks without any complication, though, in children, the lump caused by the callus may be visible for several months. It is important, when applying the triangular sling for this or any other reason, to make sure that it is sufficiently tight for the elbow to be flexed just above a right-angle, to encourage venous return from the hand and discourage stiffness of the fingers. These fractures produce a mass of callus which resolves slowly over a prolonged period. If such a lump would be unacceptable for cosmetic reasons, the patient may be confined to bed, lying on a sandbag between the shoulders, for a period of 4 weeks.

Fracture of the upper end of the humerus occurs in 2 sites: either across the surgical neck or at the base of the greater tuberosity. The former is usually impacted and rarely requires manipulation; a triangular sling is sufficient immobilization. Attempts to reduce a fracture of the greater tuberosity by immobilizing the arm in plaster of Paris in 90° of abduction are now rarely used. Non-union of this fracture is unknown; a triangular sling to rest the arm is all that is required and the patient is referred to the Fracture Clinic.

Fractures of the scapula may be difficult to see on X-ray but fortunately symptomatic treatment — a triangular sling to rest the shoulder — is the correct treatment. Fractures of the scapula only assume importance when they involve the glenoid fossa, because of the risk of subsequent stiffness and pain in the shoulder joint. When the coracoid process is fractured it may require internal fixation to achieve a satisfactory result. Do not forget that fractures of the ribs may underlie the fractured scapula.

Joint lesions

Dislocation of the shoulder joint is a common condition and its reduction is one of the most frequent manipulations the emergency doctor is required to perform. In elderly subjects the humeral head dislocates anteriorly (through the antero-inferior or weakest part of the capsule) and comes to lie in a sub-coracoid position. In young adults the capsule and labrum are stripped off the glenoid process of the scapula, again allowing the humeral head to travel medially into the sub-coracoid

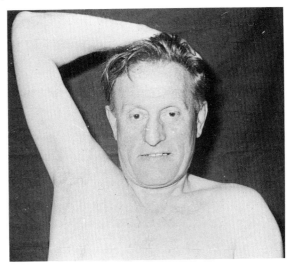

Figure 10.6.   Patient with a luxatio erecta dislocation of the shoulder joint

position. Very rarely the dislocation occurs with the arm elevated and the humeral head becomes fixed in a sub-glenoid position. The patient then comes to hospital in considerable pain, with his arm held vertically upwards — the luxatio erecta position (*Figure 10.6*).

Finally, the dislocation may be posterior. This is rare and because the humeral head cannot displace medially it may not be obvious clinically and only a slight incongruity is detectable on the antero-posterior X-ray. An axial film is required to demonstrate the full extent of the damage (*Figure 10.7*).

Manipulation

For patients with a luxatio erecta or with a posterior dislocation, manipulation is simple and can be done under intravenous analgesia. Entonox possibly supplemented with 10 mg of Diazepam is usually sufficient to allow the traction and rotation of the arm which is required to slip the humeral head back over the lip of the glenoid labrum and into the glenoid fossa.

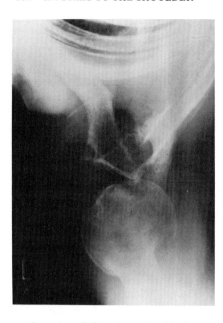

Figure 10.7.   Axial view of a posterior   dislocation   of   the shoulder

Anterior dislocations in elderly patients can frequently be reduced under intravenous analgesia, but the young adult normally requires a general anaesthetic and possibly a muscle relaxant to facilitate reduction. In elderly patients, if an attempt at reduction under analgesia is not immediately successful it must not be repeated until they too can have the benefit of a general anaesthetic and muscle relaxant.

The classic methods of reducing an anterior dislocation of the shoulder joint are attributed to Hippocrates and to Kocher. The latter is preferable and the Hippocratic method is only indicated if Kocher's manoeuvre has been unsuccessful.

There are 4 steps to Kocher's manoeuvre and they should be *performed gently, unhurriedly but firmly, in sequence.*

First movement.   An assistant (standing at the head of the patient), locks his hands in the patient's axilla. The surgeon stands on the affected side and takes hold of the wrist of the dislocated limb with one hand and gently bends the elbow to a right-angle. The other hand is now placed on the forearm, just below the elbow, and starts to press the limb distally. The pressure is gradually increased and the head of the humerus starts to move downwards towards the rent in the antero-inferior part of the capsule. This movement is often felt by the assistant's hands in the axilla.

Second movement.   When the head has moved downwards, external rotation through 70–90° is gently applied to the arm to overcome the spasm in the sub-scapularis muscle. The surgeon must maintain the traction during this manoeuvre and this is best achieved by taking small steps backwards in a semi-circle.

Third movement.   Still maintaining downward traction and external rotation, the point of the elbow is now adducted across the patient's chest. This movement levers the head of the humerus over the lip of the glenoid labrum.

Fourth movement.   Relaxing traction, the forearm is now internally rotated to be across the patient's chest thus rolling the humeral head into the glenoid fossa.

Signs of completion of the reduction

As the head of the humerus slips back into the glenoid cavity, a click or jerk is usually noticed by both surgeon and assistant. In many reductions the assistant's hands form a fulcrum around which the head is levered back into position during the second part of the manoeuvre, making parts 3 and 4 superfluous. Clinical examination will now confirm that the shoulder has regained its normal rounded contour and the humeral head can no longer be palpated in the axilla. The final proof is by X-ray examination and if there is any doubt this should be done before a general anaesthetic is terminated.

Very occasionally one has to resort to the more crude Hippocratic manoeuvre which consists of applying traction on the arm with a stockinged foot pressing on the medial wall of the axilla. This may be a more effective method but if care is not taken, it can subject the brachial plexus to direct pressure which may result in nerve damage.

After treatment

It is very important to understand the distinct difference between the anterior dislocation in the young adult and that in the elderly patient. The former, often resulting from rugby or football, involves stripping the glenoid labrum off the bone. For this to heal after the reduction, the arm must be fixed to the chest wall by a triangular sling worn under the clothes and not removed for 3 weeks. Following this, the arm should not be abducted above a right-angle for a further 3 weeks. If this rigorous treatment is not followed then recurrent dislocation is more likely and once it occurs further dislocations are extremely probable and eventually surgical treatment will be necessary. For the elderly patient all that is required is a triangular sling worn outside the clothes for 5 to 7 days until the pain settles; graded active exercises should then be encouraged to prevent joint stiffness.

Contra-indications to closed manipulation of the dislocated shoulder

In two circumstances manipulation should not be attempted in the emergency room.

The first is when the dislocation is complicated by a fracture of the neck of the humerus because any attempt at manipulation risks displacing the fracture rather than reducing the dislocation. Patients with this complication should be admitted to hospital where an orthopaedic surgeon can perform the manipulation under radiological control and proceed to an open operation if necessary.

The second contra-indication is in the patient whose dislocation happened 5 or more days ago. These are usually elderly patients for whom the pain of dislocation was not particularly severe and they wait a week or so to see if the shoulder will recover without resorting to medical treatment. These patients should all be referred to an orthopaedic surgeon. Some of them may have a successful manipulation, some may be treated by open reduction but for many of them, considering their age, general health and poor physique, it will be decided to leave the shoulder in the dislocated position. Infrequently a patient may be seen with a fresh injury superimposed on a long-standing dislocation which may have been present for many years. Closed reduction will be impossible and should not be attempted.

Acromio-clavicular dislocation

The outer end of the clavicle is displaced upwards, because of rupture of the coraco-clavicular ligaments, and projects as an obvious lump under the skin. In the past, treatment has consisted of applying strapping over a felt pad (Robert Jones technique), or of open operation. There is no evidence that the results from these methods are any better than from simply supporting the arm in a triangular sling for some 3 weeks to allow the ligaments to heal spontaneously. The prominence of the outer end of the clavicle will slowly recede as the ligaments heal.

Sterno-clavicular dislocation

This is a rare injury. If the deformity is not very great it can be left to correct itself spontaneously. If it is more marked, the inner end of the clavicle can be pushed back into place under a general anaesthetic and an attempt made to hold it in place by applying strapping over a felt pad. The results of this manipulation are unpredictable and occasionally surgical reconstruction may be considered at a later stage.

SOFT TISSUE LESIONS AROUND THE SHOULDER

These are common and although many of the conditions are not really appropriate for examination and treatment in an Emergency Department, the patients come because the symptoms are disturbing their sleep and interfering with their work. They all expect that an X-ray examination will produce an immediate diagnosis but, apart from revealing the occasional patient with calcification in the supraspinatus tendon, its only value is to exclude localized bone disease. The history and especially the physical examination are much more important in making a diagnosis and deciding treatment. Patients should first of all be divided into those who have had a definite recent injury and those whose symptoms have either come on insidiously or are more severe than can be explained by any recent minor trauma.

Patients with a recent injury

These patients have either suffered a simple sprain or contusion, or have torn a muscle or tendon. The former will have generalized pain and tenderness aggravated by movements, the latter will have localized pain and tenderness, certain precise movements being either painful or impossible. As early surgical repair is only usually considered for complete tears of the supraspinatus tendon, for most patients treatment in the first 2 weeks consists of rest and relief of pain. A triangular sling to support the arm and, if necessary, analgesic tablets should be prescribed. Electrotherapy to disperse the oedema is also widely used and in recent years we have found treatment with Diapulse to be a most effective method of relieving the pain and so allowing early mobilization.

After 2 weeks of this treatment, patients with a simple sprain or contusion should have made a full recovery. Further examination of patients with a muscle or tendon tear will now reveal a precise localized area of tenderness. This will be in 1 of 4 sites:

1. Over the point of the shoulder in relation to the supraspinatus tendon.
2. Over the long head of biceps lying in the bicipital groove on the antero-lateral aspect of the shoulder.
3. In front of the shoulder between the coracoid process and the lesser tubercle.
4. Behind the shoulder.

The latter two sites are related to the rotator cuff or tendons; an injection of hydrocortisone and local anaesthetic into the appropriate area will often relieve their symptoms. If necessary the injection can be repeated after 2 more weeks but more than 2 injections are not recommended.

Patients without a recent injury

Symptoms in these patients are due either to localized degenerative changes or are the late results of trauma — often repeated minor trauma from abnormal use of the shoulder. Three distinct conditions, one depending on a radiological diagnosis and two on the physical examination, are described.

Calcification in the supraspinatus tendon

This is seen in middle-aged people and is often excruciatingly painful. The diagnosis is made on X-ray (*Figure 10.8*). Treatment consists of decompressing the area: inject local anaesthetic into the skin, then with a wide bore needle inject hydrocortisone and local anaesthetic into the calcified mass and attempt to withdraw the toothpaste-like material. Even if the material is too thick to come up the needle the symptoms are usually relieved and, if not a sling, analgesics and Diapulse therapy can be prescribed. Only rarely is it necessary to resort to open operation and curettage.

Painful arc syndrome

The arm is pain-free at rest but as it is abducted from 60° to 120° pain is felt over the point of the shoulder. Movement above or below this arc is painless. Sub-acromial bursitis is probably the most common cause of this symptom but it may also be seen following injury to, or degenerative changes in, the supraspinatus tendon. The treatment is the

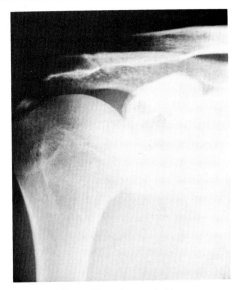

Figure 10.8. Calcification in the supraspinatus tendon

same as for recent injuries: rest in a sling, Diapulse and, if necessary, hydrocortisone and local anaesthetic injection. Analgesics are not usually indicated.

Frozen shoulder

This is a well defined syndrome which affects people around the age of 50 to 60 years. It starts with pain, felt vaguely in the deltoid region, which gradually becomes worse and interferes with sleep. The range of movement in the shoulder diminishes until only the scapulo-thoracic element of shoulder movement remains. The condition is variously described as a capsulitis or peri-arthritis and surgical exploration, if carried out, shows the capsule to be contracted and thickened. Without treatment the condition eventually resolves spontaneously but may take a year or 18 months to do so. We have found treatment with Diapulse to be valuable in reducing the pain and so enabling the patient to sleep at night. Gentle exercises can then be encouraged but the patient should not be forced to the point where he aggravates the pain.

Chronic pain referred to the shoulder from other sites

Cervical spondylosis with irritation of nerve roots, tennis elbow or occasionally compression of the median nerve in the carpal tunnel may all produce pain which is vaguely referred to the shoulder region. A careful history, physical examination and X-ray will elucidate the true cause of the symptoms.

11

Injuries to the Arm and Elbow

Injuries to the arm and elbow can be divided into:

1. Fractures.
2. Dislocations.
3. Injuries to soft tissues.

If the injury is severe, complications due to damage to vessels or nerves must be detected and these will assume priority of importance over the bony injury. When the time comes to consider the radiological appearance one cannot assume that because there is now little displacement of the bones, other structures cannot have been damaged. At the moment of fracture or dislocation there was probably a wide discursion of the bony fragments with consequent tearing of the soft tissues. Normal elastic recoil and First Aid manoeuvres will have brought the fragments almost back into line by the time the X-ray is taken — but the soft tissue damage remains.

FRACTURES

Fractures of the shaft of the humerus

As with all limb fractures it is important to check for the integrity of the circulation and peripheral nerves: look for cyanosis or swelling of the forearm and hand; feel the radial pulse. In fractures of the middle third of the humerus check especially for damage to the radial nerve by asking the patient to extend the wrist and fingers. For fractures at the lower end of the humerus or dislocation of the elbow, inability to flex the index finger when 'making a fist' indicates damage to the median nerve; inability to abduct and adduct the fingers while they are in extension implies damage to the ulnar nerve. The median and ulnar nerve injuries will be confirmed by loss of sensation on the appropriate part of the palmar aspect of the hand and fingers. Radial nerve sensory

110

innervation is very variable but when present it at least supplies the dorsum of the first web, between thumb and index.

Early manipulation of fractures of the shaft of the humerus is rarely necessary. If a collar and cuff sling is applied the weight of the arm gradually pulls the bony fragments into line. Plaster of Paris, if used, should only be applied as a slab on the outer aspect of the arm to protect it from further injury. A full arm cast is contra-indicated; not only is it unnecessary but it adds the risk of circulatory occlusion if swelling occurs within the cast. After the initial treatment the patient is referred to an Orthopaedic Clinic for supervision until the fracture is healed in about 6 weeks' time.

Supra-condylar fracture of the humerus

This is a childhood fracture resulting from a fall on the out-stretched hand. The humerus breaks just above the condyles and the lower fragment is driven backwards stretching the brachial artery over the lower end of the upper fragment (*Figure 11.1*). This fracture is the most common cause of arterial occlusion in the upper limb, therefore always check the radial pulse before and after manipulation.

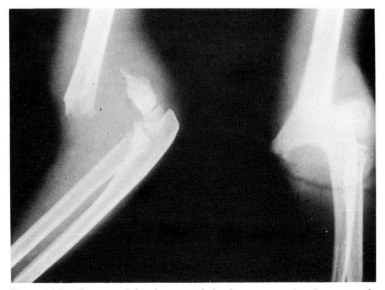

Figure 11.1. Supra-condylar fracture of the humerus causing damage to the brachial artery

Manipulation, requiring an operator and an assistant, must always be performed under a general anaesthetic. The assistant takes hold of the forearm and pulls distally with the elbow flexed at about 30°. If the lower end of the upper fragment has become impaled in the fibres of brachialis muscle it will be freed by this manoeuvre. It is then available to receive the lower fragment as this is pushed forward by the operator standing behind the arm and using his thumb to restore alignment. Perfect re-alignment on the lateral view is less essential than on the antero-posterior view where an imperfect reduction will result in a permanent deformity of the normal 'carrying angle' of the forearm.

After reduction the arm is fixed in a collar and cuff sling at an angle which does not occlude the radial pulse. There is still a risk of circulatory obstruction occurring due to swelling developing after the manipulation. Consequently, all these children should remain in hospital overnight for regular supervision of the circulation. If these precautionary steps are taken the feared complication of Volkmann's ischaemic contracture will be avoided.

Fracture of the lateral condyle of the humerus

This is a childhood fracture. Once the epicondyle and epiphysis of the capitulum have broken free the fragment usually rotates and cannot be reduced by closed manipulation. Also, accurate reconstitution of the articular surface of the elbow joint is so important that open reduction and fixation are usually required.

Fracture of the olecranon process of the ulna

This fracture is usually due to direct violence resulting in the proximal inch of the ulnar being broken off, the fracture line passing into the elbow joint. If the triceps expansion is still intact there will be minimal displacement and a triangular sling for 2 to 3 weeks is the only treatment required. More often the expansion is torn and the triceps tendon, which is inserted into the olecranon process, pulls the fragment of bone away from the rest of the ulna. Bony continuity can then only be restored by an open operation using a screw to re-position the fragment.

Fracture of the head or neck of the radius

This fracture is due to a fall on the out-stretched hand and is seen in both children and adults. Force is transmitted up the forearm driving the head of the radius against the capitulum and either the outer portion of the head breaks off or the bone breaks just below the head across the neck. Pain and tenderness are felt on the lateral side of the elbow joint and movement is restricted and painful. If the standard X-ray views do not show a fracture, further films should be taken with the radial head rotated. If there is minimal displacement, or the fracture can be reduced by a closed manipulation, a collar and cuff sling is prescribed. If a closed reduction is impossible or unsuccessful, open reduction is indicated otherwise there will be permanent impairment of elbow function and eventually osteo-arthritic changes.

Avulsed medial epicondyle of the humerus

This condition is not uncommon in children and is of little importance unless the epicondyle has been pulled into the elbow joint (*Figure 11.2*). If this occurs, manipulation under anaesthetic should be left to an

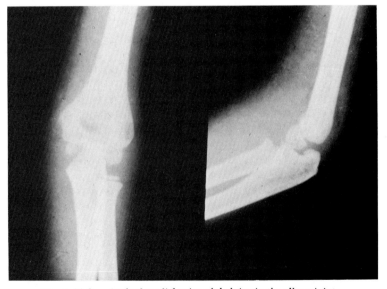

Figure 11.2.   Avulsed medial epicondyle lying in the elbow joint

orthopaedic surgeon who can proceed immediately to open operation and internal fixation if his manipulation is unsuccessful. Damage to the ulnar nerve may complicate this injury.

Interpretation of X-rays of the elbow

In the growing child, when the elbow region is 'full of epiphyses' it may be difficult to decide if a fracture is present. This dilemma is solved by taking an X-ray of the opposite, uninjured elbow which must be placed in the same degree of flexion and prono-supination to produce identical films for comparison.

DISLOCATIONS

Dislocation of the elbow joint

A patient with a recent, backward dislocation of the elbow joint should have the dislocation reduced as quickly as possible before reactionary swelling makes the reduction more difficult. If, for one reason or another, the patient cannot be given a general anaesthetic within an hour of arriving at hospital then the manipulation should be performed under intravenous analgesia or entonox. A stoical patient may even prefer to have the reduction performed without analgesia.

Method of reduction

A surgeon and an assistant are required. The surgeon stands by the patient's shoulder, facing towards the patient's feet. He picks up the arm gently with both hands, the fingers encircle the arm just above the elbow and both thumbs are placed on the tip of the olecranon process. Meanwhile, the assistant takes hold of the patient's wrist and pulls gently in the line of the deformity. Apart from exerting this gentle traction the assistant takes no other part in the manoeuvre. Pressing with his thumbs, the surgeon now pushes the olecranon over the curve of the trochlea and back into place. The gentle traction exerted by the assistant prevents the elbow flexing as the pressure is exerted by the surgeon and is an essential part of the manoeuvre. The arm is now immobilized in a collar and cuff sling, with the elbow in full flexion or as much flexion as is possible without occluding the radial artery. A check X-ray is taken to confirm the reduction and to display any associated fractures. The radial pulse must be carefully observed during the patient's stay in hospital and advice given to return immediately if the pain increases or the fingers change colour.

After treatment

It is important to explain to the patient that the elbow must remain at rest, in the sling for 3 weeks to give time for the injured tissues to heal. The patient can, and must, exercise his fingers but the elbow must remain immobilized. Plaster of Paris is not recommended because there is often considerable swelling after the reduction and a rigid cast could result in peripheral ischaemia. After 3 weeks the swelling has subsided and the sling can be discarded. The patient is warned that full extension of the elbow will not return for some weeks or months; he can practise flexion exercises but must allow full extension to return without help. Any attempt to force extension will retard the progress. Physiotherapy cannot help, and passive exercises will only serve to hinder or prevent recovery. The patient should be seen at weekly intervals and, if it is found that he has lost full flexion, a further week's rest in a sling must be prescribed. The only consolation to offer the patient is that full or almost full movement will return eventually, provided myositis ossificans does not develop.

Pulled elbow

This condition is found in young children from the ages of about 1 to 3 years and is not uncommon. The child is brought by the mother with the complaint of pain in the arm and a refusal or reluctance to use it. There is often a typical history that the child has fallen and was rescued by the mother pulling him up by the affected arm. Examination of the limb shows no swelling and an X-ray shows no abnormality. It is believed that the lesion is caused by a small subluxation of the head of the radius at the upper radio-ulnar joint.

Reduction of this subluxation is simple. One thumb is placed firmly on the head of the radius anteriorly. The forearm is held at the wrist and gently rotated through a full range while maintaining pressure over the radial head. As full rotation is reached, a click is felt by the thumb over the head of the radius. As soon as the child has recovered from the aggrieved surprise at this manoeuvre, he uses the arm normally and no further treatment is required.

INJURIES TO SOFT TISSUES

Myositis ossificans

This rare but serious complication must be suspected if the range of movement diminishes rather than increases during the recovery period. If it is present, a lateral X-ray of the elbow will show a hazy shadow anterior and proximal to the joint in the region of brachialis muscle. If this shadow is seen, the elbow must be fixed in flexion in a collar and cuff sling and the degree of flexion must be increased at bi-weekly visits for 6 weeks. At the end of this time the shadow will probably have disappeared, or certainly ceased to grow, and careful mobilization can begin again. If this regimen is followed there can still be a successful outcome.

Traumatic effusion into the elbow joint

Many patients have elbow injuries which are less severe than those discussed so far. They may not come to hospital until 1 or 2 days after the accident. Their main complaint is of loss of movement rather than pain. It may be found on physical examination that they can only flex from 30° to 90° and pronosupination is also restricted. All these patients require an X-ray. Fractures of the condyles of the humerus or the head of the radius may only be detected after careful scrutiny and study of a comparable X-ray of the opposite elbow. If no fracture is present there may still be an effusion into the joint. A useful guide to making this diagnosis is 'the fat-pad sign'. The pad of fat which normally lies flat on the anterior shaft of the humerus is raised like a pennant flag when there

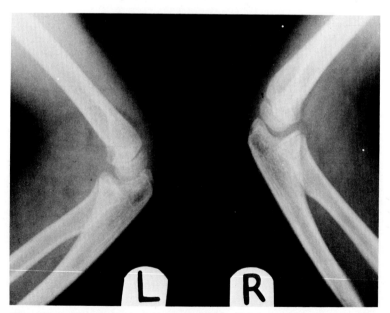

Figure 11.3.   Positive fat-pad sign indicating an effusion into the left elbow joint. Note the dark shadows projecting anteriorly from the left humerus just proximal to the elbow joint (the right elbow is shown for comparison)

is an effusion in the joint (*Figure 11.3*). Such patients still require careful management. Myositis ossificans or fibrosis of the capsule may still occur if the joint is not adequately immobilized in the early stage. A collar and cuff sling is applied under the clothes, to keep the elbow at rest until the swelling and tenderness have disappeared. This may take 2 weeks and must be followed by the same careful regimen described above for dislocation of the elbow.

Many of these injuries occur in children and their parents are naturally anxious as to when they can return to school. There is no reason why they should not attend school with the arm in a sling. When the sling has been removed, the co-operation of the teacher should be enlisted to keep the child away from violent games or compulsory physical training; games should be avoided until full movement, or almost full movement is restored. If the elbow does not improve outside interference should be suspected.

Olecranon bursitis

Swelling of the olecranon bursa often follows a blow on the point of the elbow. Severe inflammatory changes can accompany the swelling so the condition can be divided into:

1. Inflammatory cases.
2. Non-inflammatory cases.

Inflammatory bursitis

The inflammatory swellings can vary from a tense red swelling with slight surrounding cellulitis, to a small, red swelling of the bursa surrounded by gross cellulitis with oedema reaching half-way down the forearm.

Treatment. As with inflammatory prepatella bursitis, conservative treatment is the most satisfactory. Incision into the inflamed bursa leaves a wound which is very slow to heal. If the swelling is very tense the sero-purulent fluid should be aspirated from the side of the swelling, not over the point of the elbow, using a wide-bore needle. Rest in a sling and antibiotic therapy appropriate to the infecting organism, will bring rapid relief but it may be several weeks before the induration around the bursa finally disappears.

Non-inflammatory bursitis

The non-inflammatory swellings of the bursa may follow a specific blow on the elbow, but can also follow recurrent irritation, e.g. beat elbow in miners.

Treatment.   If the swelling is very tense the fluid should be aspirated through normal skin at the side of the swelling. The swelling will probably recur within 2 to 3 days although, hopefully, not to the same degree, and the aspiration can be repeated. Firm bandaging and rest for the elbow discourages recurrence, but the bandaging is irksome and may be considered a greater disability than the original swelling. This condition will usually resolve spontaneously in time, but recurrent attacks causing inconvenience to the patient may be treated by excision of the bursa.

12

Injuries to the Forearm and Wrist

Fractures of the forearm occur frequently and fractures of the wrist are the most common of all fractures. Their recognition and early management form an important part of the work of any doctor in an Accident and Emergency Department. Thus, although with most fractures we have left the details of treatment to standard works on the subject, the early management of the Colles' fracture is described in some detail.

In addition to those patients presenting with a painful swelling around the wrist, due to a fracture, there will be a number of patients with similar symptoms but no fracture. The recognition and treatment of these soft tissue injuries is just as important to the patient.

FRACTURES IN THE FOREARM

Either due to a fall onto the out-stretched hand or to direct violence, one or both of the forearm bones may be broken. If only one bone is broken in mid-shaft then, after a moment's reflection, it must be obvious that this fracture cannot be manipulated (unless the other bone is deliberately broken − and this is not an acceptable form of treatment). The nature of the fracture varies through 4 stages.

Fracture of one bone only

1. *Greenstick fracture* − no manipulation is required. Apply a plaster of paris back slab.
2. *Undisplaced fracture* − no manipulation is required. Apply an above-elbow plaster of Paris cast.
3. *Displaced fracture* − this is most commonly seen in the middle third of the radius and, as it cannot be reduced by closed manipulation, open reduction and internal fixation is necessary.
4. *Displaced fracture with overlapping of the bone ends* − overlapping, or shortening of the broken bone can only occur if the

other, intact bone has been dislocated either at the elbow (as in the Monteggia fracture) or at the wrist (as in the Galeazzi fracture). Clearly, to demonstrate this the radiograph must include the elbow and wrist joints. Treatment is by open operation.

Fractures of both bones

1. *Greenstick fractures* — if angulated, the deformity must be corrected by a manipulation under a general anaesthetic. Pressure should be applied until a slight 'crack' is felt or heard; until this 'crack' occurs the bones will spring back into their position of deformity after the grip is released. Aplly an above-elbow plaster of Paris cast (*see below*).
2. *Undisplaced fractures* — no manipulation is required. Apply an above-elbow plaster of Paris cast (*see below*).
3. *Displaced fractures* — when both bones of the forearm are broken and displaced their reduction requires skill and experience. The radiological appearance may suggest that the reduction will be relatively easy, but this is rarely true. In the child, 'periosteal splinting' makes it necessary to exaggerate the deformity to almost 90° before the lower fragment can be brought in line. In the adult, even if a good reduction is obtained it is difficult to maintain and internal fixation is often necessary. Consequently, when faced with a patient with displaced fractures of both forearm bones, the inexperienced doctor will be well advised to seek advice and help from a trained surgeon.

Plaster of Paris casts for forearm fractures

The degree of prono-supination in which the forearm is immobilized in an above-elbow plaster cast depends on the level of the fractures.

1. *Fractures in the upper third of the forearm* — apply the cast with the forearm in supination, the palm of the hand being uppermost to allow for the supinating pull of biceps tendon on the upper element of the fracture.
2. *Fractures in the middle third of the forearm* — apply the cast with the forearm in a neutral position, the thumb being uppermost. Pronator teres is now balancing the pull of biceps on the upper fragment.
3. *Fractures in the lower third of the forearm* — apply the cast with the forearm in pronation, the back of the hand being uppermost, to allow for the added pull of pronator quadratus.

INJURIES AROUND THE WRIST JOINT

History

The time which has elapsed since the injury occurred should be noted; the cause of the injury and the nature of the violence should also be recorded. Such notes may be of value in compensation enquiries. For instance, either of the two following notes may precede descriptions of identical injuries:

> 'Fell onto out-stretched right hand on way home from pub at 11.00 pm last night.'

or 'Slipped on oil spilt on workshop floor at 9.00 am this morning and fell onto out-stretched right hand.'

The compensation potential of the latter considerably outweighs the former.

Physical examination

This follows the standard sequence of: look, feel, move, and X-ray.

Look

The classical 'dinner-fork' deformity of the Colles' fracture (*Figure 12.1*) is often so obvious that the diagnosis can be made at this preliminary stage. Fullness of the anatomical snuff box, indicating a fracture of the radial styloid or the scaphoid, may only be appreciated by comparing the two wrists. Similarly, the swelling of a child's chubby forearm, due

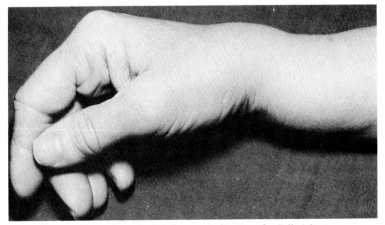

Figure 12.1.   Dinner-fork deformity indicative of a Colles' fracture

to an undisplaced Greenstick fracture of the radius, may only be obvious when the two arms are compared. Swelling or deformity will also accompany other fractures or dislocations of the carpus.

The characteristic sausage-shaped swelling of tenosynovitis extending upwards from the dorsum of the wrist for 5 to 7 cm along the line of the long tendons of the thumb is diagnostic.

Feel

Eliciting localized tenderness is of value and will be a guide to requesting and interpreting the X-rays. Tenderness in the anatomical snuff box, even in the absence of swelling, suggests a fracture of the radial styloid or scaphoid bones. In tenosynovitis, crepitus is often felt over the swelling as the patient moves the thumb or wrist. The remainder of the wrist, hand and fingers should be palpated for tenderness which the patient has not thought to mention, and any diminution in cutaneous sensation must be detected.

Move

Limited movement due to pain or stiffness in the wrist or fingers should be recorded. If there is a full range of movement there is unlikely to be any serious pathology.

X-Ray

Normally 2 views, antero-posterior and lateral are sufficient. Because of the multiplicity of the bony surfaces, it is wise to follow the outline of each one individually to avoid missing a fracture or a carpal dislocation. Particular attention must be paid to the bones in the area of tenderness. When the examination suggests that the scaphoid may be injured, 4 views are necessary to be sure to demonstrate a fracture across the waist of the bone.

Treatment

Fractures without displacement

These, apart from a scaphoid fracture, are treated quite simply by a dorsal slab of plaster of Paris applied over 'plaster wool'. The slab must extend from the metacarpophalangeal joints upwards almost to the bend of the elbow (the edge of the slab should not dig into the arm when the elbow is flexed). The slab should be broad enough to curl over the sides of the wrist with a piece cut out from one edge to accommodate the thumb. The wet slab is fixed in place by a cotton bandage with 3 turns of the bandage going round the palm. A triangular sling is then applied with the elbow flexed just above a right-angle, so that the wrist is higher than the elbow and venous stasis in the hand will be prevented.

Patients are warned to return immediately if the fingers become blue, swollen, or painful; otherwise they attend the next Fracture Clinic by which time the reactionary swelling should have subsided and the plaster slab can be completed into a full plaster cast to be worn for 6 weeks.

Scaphoid fractures

This injury is treated by applying a full forearm cast over plaster wool. The plaster passes from just below the elbow to the heads of the meta-carpals of the fingers. On the thumb it encloses the proximal phalanx, just leaving the interphalangeal joint free. To apply this cast ask the patient to position his hand as if he were holding an orange or a cricket ball (whichever seems the more appropriate).

Occasionally patients have pain, tenderness and slight swelling in the anatomical snuff box but no fracture can be seen on the initial X-rays; they should be treated in a scaphoid cast as if a fracture were present. After 14 days remove the cast and repeat the X-rays. If there is still no fracture to be seen they can be reassured and discharged. If a fracture is now evident, then 2 weeks have been saved and the risk of further trauma in the intervening period, producing an aggravating injury and making avascular necrosis more likely, has been avoided.

Colles' fracture

This is the most common of all fractures and is especially prevalent in post-menopausal women. It is a fracture in the lower inch of the radius, usually with dorsal angulation of the distal fragment, caused by a fall on the out-stretched hand. Most Accident Departments in Britain can recall days when the first frost of winter brought 20 or 30 or more such patients within the space of a few hours.

The clinical picture of the 'dinner-fork' deformity has already been mentioned (*Figure 12.1*). Close scrutiny of the typical X-ray appearance

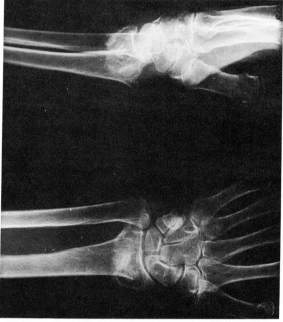

Figure 12.2. Colles' fracture. The lower fragment of the radius is displaced backwards, rotated backwards and impacted. It is also laterally displaced and there is a fracture of the ulnar styloid process

will show that there is a possible total of 6 different aspects of the bony injury, some or all of which will be present in any one patient:

1. Impaction of the lower fragment into the shaft of the radius.
2. Dorsal displacement.
3. Dorsal rotation.
4. Lateral displacement.
5. Comminution of the distal fragment with the fracture line entering the wrist joint.
6. An associated fracture of the ulnar styloid process (*Figure 12.2*).

Reduction of the fracture

This is performed under general anaesthesia or a regional block. If the following steps are carried out in order and in their entirety the reduction and fixation should always be successful.

Disimpact the fracture

An assistant holds the arm just above the elbow. The surgeon holds the patient's fingers in one hand and the thumb in the other. They pull in opposite directions, the younger the patient, the stronger the pull required. The movement as the bony fragments are disimpacted is usually felt and may sometimes be heard.

Correct the remaining deformity

To do this, the surgeon stands inside the abducted arm with his back to the prone body of the patient.

1. Place the patient's wrist in pronation. For a fracture of the right wrist the surgeon places the thenar eminence of his left hand over the displaced lower end of the radius with his fingers and thumb encircling the ulnar border of the wrist.
2. The surgeon then places his right hand beneath the lower end of the forearm with his hypothenar eminence just proximal to the

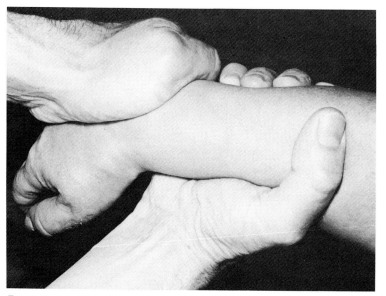

Figure 12.3.   After disimpacting a Colles' fracture by traction, use this grip to correct the dorsal displacement and rotation, and to produce ulnar deviation at the wrist

line of the fracture. The fingers of this hand curl round the ulnar border of the lower forearm.

3. Using the hypothenar eminence of the right hand as a fulcrum, the surgeon now hyper-extends his left wrist as he presses down with his left thenar eminence on the lower fragment of the radius, forcing it downwards, forwards and ulnarwards all in one movement (*Figure 12.3*).

Note: no particular attention is paid to the ulnar styloid process if it is fractured.

Immobilize the fracture

Once reduced, the fracture is then immobilized using a plaster of Paris back slab in the way already described for undisplaced fractures. While the slab is being bandaged on the limb the surgeon holds the patient's fingers in one hand and the thumb in the other and applies gentle traction by leaning backwards. The patient's wrist will thus fall into the natural position of ulnar deviation. As soon as the slab has been fixed, the surgeon returns to the inner side of the arm and re-applies the grip used for the manipulation — but without applying any pressure — until the plaster is set hard. An X-ray is now taken to check the reduction. Apart from restoring alignment it is important to confirm on the lateral view that the angle between the lower end of the radius and the proximal carpal bones is once again $5-10°$ forward of the vertical (*Figure 12.4*).

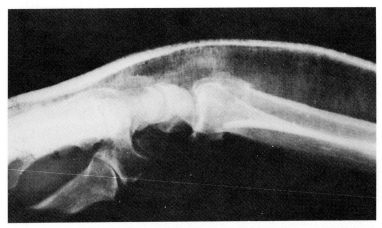

Figure 12.4.   Colles' fracture reduced and immobilized by a plaster of Paris back slab

After treatment

A triangular sling is applied with the elbow flexed above a right-angle and the patient warned to return immediately if the fingers become painful, blue or swollen. The patient is also given an appointment for the next Fracture Clinic when, if all is well, the slab will be converted into a full cast.

Other fractures and dislocations around the wrist

Smith's fracture

This is 'the reverse of a Colles' fracture', the distal fragment being displaced ventrally instead of dorsally. The median nerve is consequently at risk and it is especially important to check its integrity both before and after the manipulation. When performing the manipulation, after disimpaction, the surgeon stands on the outer side of the forearm with his lower hand on the ventral side of the patient's wrist and the more proximally positioned hand on the dorsum of the lower forearm. The wrist should be immobilized in supination in an above-elbow cast.

Fracture-dislocation of the lower radial epiphysis

This occurs in children and is treated in the same way as a Colles' fracture except that no preliminary traction is necessary because there is no impaction.

Dislocations

Dislocation of the wrist joint is a rare injury requiring very considerable force. More frequently, although still rare, a dislocation occurs through the carpal bones leaving the lunate, and sometimes half the scaphoid, still articulating with the radius. These perilunar or trans-scaphoid dislocations can be difficult to reduce, and carry a considerable morbidity. They should be managed by an experienced surgeon, but the junior doctor must be able to recognize them when they occur. The secret is to follow the outline of each of the carpal bones in turn and any incongruity between adjacent bones implies a dislocation. Remember that the patient, almost certainly, has another uninjured wrist available for comparison.

Soft tissue injuries around the wrist

Sprain of the wrist joint

This is a dangerous diagnosis to make without adequate radiological examination. If the symptoms suggest a fracture even though none is seen on X-ray a forearm plaster of Paris cast is still recommended. When it is removed after 2 weeks repeat the X-ray. If it is still negative, despite symptoms still being present, apply elastoplast strapping for a further 2 weeks; this can be followed, if necessary, by an elastic support or crêpe bandage.

Traumatic ganglion of the wrist

Following minor trauma some patients develop a tender, tense, cystic swelling about the size of a pea. This is due to herniation of the synovial membrane of the wrist joint through the fibrous capsule. They seem to produce symptoms and distress to the patient out of all proportion to their size. Treatment is eventually by aspiration, but it is advisable to apply elastoplast strapping to the wrist for a couple of weeks first, to give time for the neck of the sac to be sealed off, otherwise the swelling may recur as soon as the fluid is removed. Only if and when this treatment fails to give a lasting cure, should open excision be used.

Tenosynovitis of the wrist

This condition presents in 2 forms, wet and dry. The wet variety, often associated with rheumatoid disease, may follow a direct blow or an isolated wrench of the wrist, but is more often caused by unusual, repetitive use of the wrist. A bank clerk cutting the garden hedge or a manual worker returning to work after illness or an industrial dispute are likely canditates. An effusion develops in the sheath surrounding abductor pollucis longus and extensor pollucis brevis tendons and is obvious as a sausage shaped swelling passing obliquely up the back of the forearm for 5 to 7 cm from the radial side of the wrist. Palpation often elicits crepitus as the patient flexes and extends the thumb.

The dry variety of tenosynovitis, more precisely described as a tendovaginitis or De Quervain's disease, is a particular problem of people whose daily work involves repetitive use of the wrist. There is pain and tenderness in the region of Lister's tubercle on the back of the wrist and crepitus may be felt on movement of the wrist.

Treatment. This is initially conservative. The synovitis with an effusion often responds well to an injection of hydrocortisone and rest for 10 days. The tendovaginitis is more difficult to cure. Hydrocortisone and strapping or even plaster of Paris immobilization are recommended as an initial treatment, but many patients are only relieved of their symptoms after surgical decompression of the tendon sheaths. Even then it may be necessary for some of them to change their occupation to avoid recurrent attacks.

13

Hand Injuries

The hand is the most frequently injured part of the body. Patients with hand injuries may form up to 10 per cent of the total case load of an Accident and Emergency Department. The importance for daily living of this complex, combined motor and sensory member is rarely appreciated until it is injured or mutilated. For most people, wage earning, running a home, and the majority of recreational pleasures depend on the integrity of their hands. Consequently, it is essential that every doctor working in an Accident Department be competent in the management of hand injuries. He must be able to make a comprehensive diagnosis, and understand clearly which conditions he may treat and which he should refer to a specialist hand surgeon.

After discussing the importance of the history and the physical examination, treatment of injuries to the various structures in the hand will be described. It is important to remember that these individual injuries do not necessarily occur in isolation and any one structure intimately affects another. The hand must be seen as an entity throughout the whole period of injury and rehabilitation.

HISTORY

The cause of the injury and the time at which it occurred must be noted. The nature of the trauma may suggest the possibility of foreign bodies being embedded in the wound or, as in the case of a hand trapped between moving rollers, that the damage to the skin and subcutaneous tissue will be much more extensive than is at first apparent. The reduction of a dislocated interphalangeal joint, performed on the sportsfield, is important to record because although physical signs may be minimal and the X-ray will be normal, there can be pain and stiffness for 2 to 3 weeks.

The circumstances in which the injury occurred are important, and should be recorded before they become embellished by frequent repetition. Industrial injuries may eventually result in medical evidence being required for litigation. Injuries sustained in the course of a crime may subsequently have to be described in a medico-legal statement or in a Court of Law, and if the details were not recorded at the time it will be impossible to recall them accurately at a later date. Self-inflicted injuries, serious though they may be, indicate that the patient has problems which go deeper than the physical wound and for which they are crying out for help.

Finally, this period of history-taking is invaluable for establishing rapport, for getting in touch with the patient. One must enquire as to which is the patient's dominant hand, and ask about his work, recreation and hobbies, and assess his attitude to his injury, because these factors may possibly influence the treatment and will definitely have a bearing on the success of the patient's rehabilitation.

PHYSICAL EXAMINATION

This follows the classical steps of: look, feel, move and X-ray.

Look

Inspect the hand for bruising, swelling, deformity, inflammation and wounds, and examine both sides of the hand. Patients can be so perverse as to show you a wound on the palmar surface and not think it necessary to mention that the extensor surface is also injured.

It will often be possible, by inspection alone, to diagnose a dislocated interphalangeal joint or, in a dangling finger, to suspect that the flexor tendons have been divided; but the patient still merits a full examination of the hand.

Feel

Approach the injured hand gently, just as one does when palpating the abdomen. Feel for tenderness, swelling, crepitus and sensory loss. To test for anaesthesia it is essential to obscure the patient's vision and, in the recently injured hand, it is preferable to stroke it lightly with your index finger or a piece of cotton wool rather than inflict further trauma by using a pin or needle.

Move

Movements are either 'active', which the patient performs himself, or 'passive' which you do to him. Always start with active movements first. Test the fingers for extension and flexion, including flexion of the distal interphalangeal joints. Ask the patient to spread the fingers in abduction.

Examine the thumb for flexion, extension, adduction and abduction. Record any loss of full movement. Where there is loss of active movement, gently apply passive movement. If there is a fracture or dislocation, this will be difficult and painful. Conversely, if the deficit is due to nerve or tendon damage, passive movement will still be possible. There are some patients with severely crushed or mutilated hands in whom this precise distinction is not possible and they will require assessment by an experienced hand surgeon.

By this time it should be possible to form a definite opinion about damage to the major nerves:

1. *Radial nerve damage* above the elbow, causes a drop wrist and loss of extension of the fingers and a variable patch of anaesthesia centred over the dorsum of the first web.
2. *Ulnar nerve damage* causes paralysis of the intrinsic muscles of the hand, with a loss of abduction and adduction of the extended fingers. True opposition of thumb to index will also be absent. Anaesthesia usually involves the ulnar border of the palm, the little and half the ring fingers.
3. *High median nerve lesion*, in the region of the elbow: the patient cannot flex the index finger and has little or no flexion in the middle finger. He cannot abduct the thumb and has anaesthesia usually involving the palmar aspect of the radial 3½ fingers.
4. *Low median nerve injury*. Division of the median nerve at the wrist is the most common of peripheral nerve injuries. It is caused by lacerations on a pane of glass or by self-inflicted knife wounds. The only motor deficit from this injury is abduction of the thumb. To test for this the hand must be flat on a table, palmar side upwards, and the patient must attempt to point his thumb to the ceiling. All other movements in the fingers and thumb will be unaffected. The area of anaesthesia is the same as in the high median nerve lesion.

Very occasionally when a patient has sustained a partial lesion of a nerve, the physical signs will be less precise.

X-Ray

Antero-posterior and oblique views of the hand will reveal fractures or dislocation and any pre-existing abnormality of the bones or joints. Foreign bodies will usually be obvious. Metal stands out clearly, glass usually contains sufficient lead to make a definite shadow but plastic objects may be difficult to identify.

TREATMENT

Injuries to the skin and subcutaneous tissue

The principles of treatment are described in Chapter 18, and the management of the burned hand is discussed in Chapter 19. However, the hand poses certain problems because it is so frequently exposed to injury and these merit separate description.

Avulsed finger nail

If the nail has been completely ripped off, apply a non-adhesive dressing for a week to 10 days until the nail bed is re-epithelialized. Eventually a new nail will grow. If the nail has only been partially avulsed, leave it *in situ* as a protective biological dressing. As the new nail grows it will expel the old one.

Sub-ungual haematoma

This is a common painful condition. The pain can be instantly relieved by trephining the nail with a hot wire to release the blood which is trapped beneath it (*Figure 13.1*).

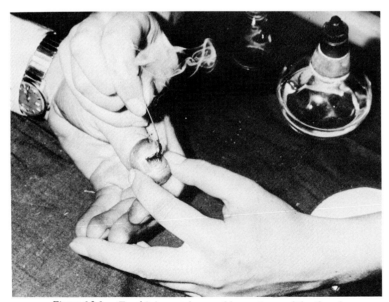

Figure 13.1.   Trephining a sub-ungual haematoma of the thumb

Local skin loss

When the wound edges cannot be brought together without tension, small partial thickness skin grafts can be taken from the thigh under a local anaesthetic, and used to cover the defect. Although they take well, as with all free grafts, they do not gain any sensory innervation. Often in the hand, bone, tendon or joint capsule are exposed in the wound and then a full thickness skin graft is required. If the area to be covered does not exceed 2 cm in any direction, a free graft can be taken from the forearm and the donor site closed by undermining the edges and performing a primary suture. Donor and graft site should then be dressed and left undisturbed for 8 to 10 days. If the area to be covered is more than 2 cm across in any direction, then a skin flap is required and the junior doctor will be wise to seek the advice of an experienced surgeon. Cross-finger flaps, thenar flaps, pectoral flaps, cross-arm flaps, inguinal flaps and neurovascular flaps may each be of value in appropriate circumstances.

Injuries involving rings

If the patient has a ring proximal to the injury it must be removed. If this is difficult and the skin is intact, soap may serve as a lubricant; failing this a ring cutter must be used (*Figure 13.2*). People working with machinery should not wear rings (*Figure 13.3*).

Traumatic amputations

Not involving the terminal phalanx

In a child, apply a non-adhesive dressing – the finger tip will regenerate. In the adult, primary skin closure is the treatment of choice, if it can be achieved, because it will preserve sensation at the finger tip. If this is impossible, a 'VY' advancement flap as described by Kutler is a second choice and a free full thickness graft from the forearm is a last resort, because it will result in a numb finger tip.

Involving the terminal phalanx

In the young child the finger can still be left to regenerate. In the older patient 'terminalization', in which the bone is nibbled back to allow primary skin closure without tension, is preferable. Admittedly this will

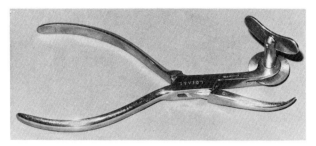

Figure 13.2.   Ring cutter for removing rings from fingers

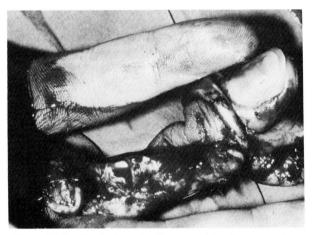

*Figure 13.3.   De-gloving of a finger resulting from a wedding
ring caught in moving machinery*

result in a short finger, but it will have good sensation. For a patient
such as a violinist, who requires a high degree of skill in his fingers, an
expert surgical opinion should be obtained before any operation is performed.

Proximal to the terminal phalanx

The finger is now too short to justify a 'plastic procedure'. The bone
should be resected back to allow primary skin closure, making sure that
the bone end is well covered by skin and subcutaneous tissue.

In the thumb

The same principles apply, but it is more important to preserve the length of the thumb as well as sensation and a neurovascular flap technique is of particular value.

Post-operatively

In all these patients the hand should be rested in a high sling to discourage oedema formation. If the sutures are non-absorbable they should be removed after 7 to 10 days and then active rehabilitation begun immediately. Ideally the patient should be back at work within 4 to 6 weeks.

Tendon injuries

Extensor tendons

Three characteristic injuries occur in the extensor mechanism of the fingers:

1. Division of a tendon in a lacerated wound.
2. Middle slip rupture producing a boutonniere deformity.
3. Avulsion of the insertion of the tendon into the terminal phalanx producing a mallet finger deformity.

The divided tendon should be repaired using a figure-of-eight non-absorbable suture followed by immobilization of the wrist and finger in

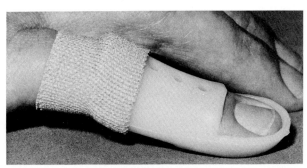

Figure 13.4.   A plastic mallet finger splint used to immobilize the distal interphalangeal joint

extension for 3 weeks. Immobilization may be achieved using either plaster of Paris or a foam padded malleable metal splint.

   Middle slip rupture is not always easy to recognize when it first occurs but as the lateral slips of the extensor mechanism prolapse to the sides of the proximal interphalangeal joint, the typical 'boutonniere' deformity develops. The sooner surgical repair is performed the better will be the result.

Mallet finger deformity is a very common problem. Although various surgical procedures are in use it is doubtful if any of them produce better results than immobilizing the distal interphalangeal joint in a 'mallet finger splint' for 6 weeks (*Figure 13.4*).

Flexor tendons

The repair of these tendons is a task for an experienced hand surgeon. In the clean, incised wound, primary repair is indicated. If it fails, a secondary procedure can be followed as is indicated when the initial injury is contused and contaminated. This consists of using a silastic rod to stimulate the growth of a new flexor sheath into which a tendon graft is subsequently introduced. If the tendon injury is associated with a fracture of the proximal phalanx and especially if the fracture involves the interphalangeal joint, amputation may be the kindest treatment. Such a decision can only be taken by an experienced surgeon after fully discussing the situation with the patient.

Nerve injuries

Division of one of the main nerves, or one or more of the branches of the median or ulnar nerve in the hand or fingers, requires primary repair by a surgeon who is experienced in the use of an operating microscope.

Vascular injuries

Similarly, modern techniques in microvascular surgery have made it possible to restore the circulation following some injuries where previously amputation was necessary. Occasionally, fingers amputated in a guillotine-type injury have been successfully re-implanted. As soon as the finger is received at the Accident Department it should be placed in a sterile (or clean) plastic bag and the bag placed in a bowl of ice.

Fractures

Metacarpals

Thumb. Because the first metacarpal is so mobile, when fractured it requires immobilization in plaster of Paris and, if this will not hold the fragments in a satisfactory position, internal fixation is indicated.

Bennett's fracture involves the carpo-metacarpal joint with a free triangular fragment on the ulnar aspect. Treatment is either by a plaster of Paris forearm cast with the thumb in full extension, or by internal fixation.

Third and fourth metacarpals.   These are naturally splinted by the second and fifth metacarpals, so a light plaster of Paris cast or even a padded bandage is all that is necessary.

Second and fifth metacarpals.   Fractures of the shaft, if stable are treated in a cast but internal fixation is more often required because of the mobility of these bones. Fracture of the neck of the fifth metacarpal is probably the most common fracture in the hand. It results from a blow delivered with a closed fist. If the angulation at the fracture exceeds 25° it should be manipulated under an anaesthetic. Then the ring and little fingers are immobilized round a roll of bandage with the metacarpophalangeal joints held at 90° for 2 to 3 weeks.

Phalanges

If the fracture is displaced it requires reduction under either a local or general anaesthetic. Then for any phalangeal fracture the treatment depends on the position in which the fracture is stable. These are, in order of preference:

1. *Stable in any position* — apply neighbour strapping for 2 weeks (*Figure 13.5*).

2. *Stable in flexion* — strap the finger and the adjacent finger round a roll of bandage for 2 to 3 weeks.

3. *Stable in extension* — strap the finger to a malleable metal splint for 2 to 3 weeks.

4. *Unstable in any position* — internal fixation.

A compound, comminuted fracture of the terminal phalanx requires excision of the displaced fragments of bone because they will not reunite and, if they are not removed, will result in a tender swollen finger end.

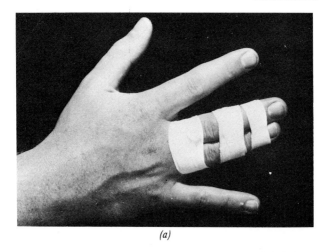

(a)

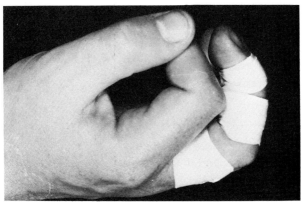

(b)

Figure 13.5. (a) and (b) Neighbour strapping for treating a stable phalangeal fracture. The uninjured finger functions as a mobile splint

Injuries to joints

Direct trauma or dislocation of a finger joint will cause an effusion in the joint and swelling around it. A period of rest for 7 to 10 days should be followed by active exercises and wax baths. Diapulse therapy is of value in reducing the pain and swelling and thereby hastening recovery,

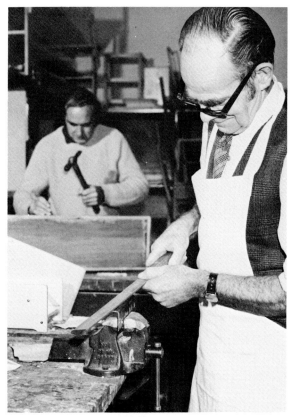

*Figure 13.6.   Occupational therapy. Hand rehabilitation for
a patient who has suffered a partial amputation of the right
index finger*

and this can be applied daily through the dressing from the day of
injury. A patient who only comes for treatment several days after the
injury may develop a 'spindle finger' in which fibroblasts invade the
swollen tissues and produce a characteristic chronic swelling which may
take several months to resolve.

REHABILITATION

Active rehabilitation must be started immediately if any of the finger
joints are stiff 10 days after skin repair, 3 weeks after tendon suture, or
as soon as a fracture is stable. The only condition in which the earliest

practical mobilization may be harmful is nerve suture. Traction applied too early to the suture line may produce scarring rather than nerve fibre regeneration.

Reference has already been made to the value of Diapulse therapy because it can be given during the period of immobilization. Wax baths and active exercises under the skilled supervision of a physiotherapist can be followed in a few days by group therapy in a hand class. Persistent stiffness or contractures may be treated by assisted exercises and corrective splinting. Occupational therapy is invaluable in preparing the patient to return to normal activities or, if this is not possible, enabling him to gain the maximum possible use from his hand (*Figure 13.6*).

14

Injuries to the Pelvic Girdle and Hips

In the Accident and Emergency Department, we see injuries to the pelvic girdle and hips presenting in 4 groups:

1. Patients with generalized pain around the pelvis and hips, usually following severe trauma.

2. Patients with pain centred around the joint following direct or indirect violence to the hip region.

3. Patients with pain over the sacrum and coccyx following a fall on the buttocks or other direct trauma.

4. Patients with a limp or pain on walking following a less severe injury some days before.

Patients in the first 2 groups are almost invariably brought into the department on a stretcher; those in the other 2 groups may walk in.

GROUP 1 –

GENERALIZED PAIN AROUND THE PELVIS

History

A severe traffic accident should always suggest that the pelvis is at risk, although the patient may not be able to describe the point of impact on the body. Blows to the perineum from falling astride a bar or the impact of a saddle are often specifically remembered.

Physical examination

When the history suggests that the pelvis is at risk, or there is a definite story of trauma to the pelvic area, examination is directed:

1. To the discovery of pain and tenderness suggesting bony injury; *and*
2. More important, to the discovery of signs suggesting injury to the bladder, urethra or other pelvic viscera.

Bony injury

Compression of the pelvis or palpation of the subcutaneous bones may produce tenderness and indicate the necessity for an X-ray examination. The whole of the pelvis is X-rayed and the outlines of all bones examined in turn for solution of the continuity. Fractures of the rami of pubis and ischium should suggest the possibility of damage to the bladder and urethra. Fractures of the wing of ilium should suggest the possibility of damage to abdominal viscera. The absence of fracture does not mean that visceral injury is not present.

Injury to the bladder, urethra or other viscera

Examine the penis for free haemorrhage from the external meatus; its presence gives evidence of damage to the urethra.

Examine the perineum for bruising and swelling. If present, this suggests the urethra may be damaged, even though external haemorrhage may not be present. If the patient has passed urine since the accident and no haematuria was present, injuries to the urethra can be ruled out. If, however, urine has not been passed, the patient should not be encouraged to do so.

Examine the abdomen for signs of tenderness suggesting rupture of the viscera (*see* Chapter 8).

Treatment

Bony injuries

Most patients with injuries to the bony ring of the pelvis will require admission to the wards for treatment. Isolated fractures of the wing of the ilium can be treated by rest in bed at home, but the decision for this form of treatment is best left to the orthopaedic surgeon.

Visceral injuries

Patients with these injuries are transferred to the beds of the general or urological wards without delay. In rupture or suspected rupture of the urethra, operation is required before extravasation occurs. If possible, the patient should therefore be discouraged from passing urine.

GROUP 2 – PAIN CENTRED ON THE HIP JOINT

History

In the elderly patient, pain in the hip following direct or indirect violence is strong presumptive evidence of fracture. There may be a delay of several days before these patients are sent to hospital, for the pain may not be so great as to demand urgent attention and these patients stay in bed after the injury and only send for a doctor when the pain does not lessen.

In the young adult, pain in the hip of such severity that movement is an agony suggests a dislocation.

Examination

In the elderly, a shortened limb, lying in external rotation, is often very obvious, and suggests a fracture of the neck of the femur (*Figure 14.1*). Where shortening of the limb is not obvious, examination of the area of the hip joint may show undue prominence of the greater trochanter or bruising of the affected side. In a number of patients, physical examination may reveal little direct evidence of the nature of the lesion and diagnosis awaits the X-ray examination.

X-Ray examination

Good quality films are essential for an accurate diagnosis (*see* Chapter 3). The A-P film must include the whole pelvis and both hip joints in order to show possible fractures of the acetabulum or adjacent rami of pubis and ischium, as well as the femoral necks. A good lateral view of the femoral neck is also necessary. Some impacted fractures of the neck of the femur are at first only obvious on the lateral view, but usually careful, repeated scrutiny of the trabeculae on the A-P view will confirm the diagnosis. The neck of the femur is a relatively common site for

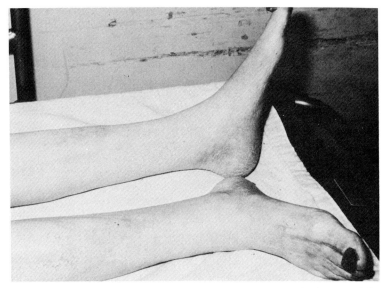

Figure 14.1.   A short, externally rotated right leg indicative of a fracture of the neck of the femur (the patient also has bilateral onychogryphosis)

pathological fractures from secondary carcinoma, and if this is suspected further physical and radiological examination may be necessary to locate the primary, for instance in breast or bronchus. Comparison of the 2 halves of the pelvis is advisable before making a firm decision that no fracture is present.

Treatment

Fractures of the neck of the femur, acetabulum or adjacent rami

These patients all require admission to hospital. No special splinting is needed for their transport to the ward; ordinary careful handling is all that is necessary.

Central dislocation of the hip

This is the usual complication of a fracture of the acetabulum and, as stated above, prompt admission to a hospital ward is indicated.

146

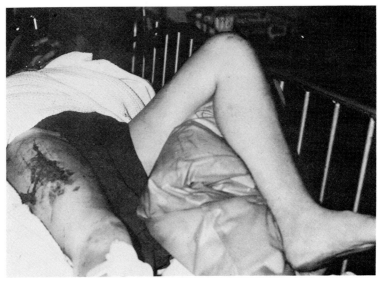

*Figure 14.2.   Anterior dislocation of the hip. Note the position in which the leg
is supported prior to reduction*

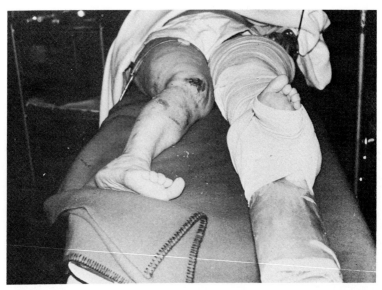

*Figure 14.3.   Posterior dislocation of the right hip. The leg is short and internally
rotated. The kiss mark on the patella indicates the point at which the force was
applied to the leg*

Anterior dislocation of the hip

This is rare, but is so painful as to justify reduction under general anaesthesia in the A & E Department, if this can be arranged promptly. The patient arrives with the hip held in flexion and abduction (*Figure 14.2*).

Posterior dislocation of the hip

This is relatively common and, when associated with more obvious fractures in the same limb, is occasionally overlooked (*Figure 14.3*). In this condition the sciatic nerve is at risk and before any manipulation is undertaken, its integrity should be confirmed by asking the patient to move his toes. To reduce the dislocation the patient must be fully relaxed under a general anaesthetic. Then, standing over the patient, the operator flexes the patient's hip and knee and applies traction to the thigh to pull the head of the femur forwards over the posterior rim of the acetabulum and into the socket. With the patient lying on the operating table this manoeuvre can be difficult and it may be necessary to lift the patient onto a mattress on the floor. If the posterior rim of the acetabulum has been fractured, the loose fragment of bone may fall into the hollow of the acetabulum and obstruct reduction of the femoral head. This situation can only be treated by an open reduction.

After manipulation a check X-ray is taken and, if the dislocation is reduced, the patient can be transported to the orthopaedic ward almost free of pain.

GROUP 3 – PAIN OVER THE SACRUM AND COCCYX

History

If the history reveals a fall onto the buttocks or a direct blow over the sacrum producing pain made worse by sitting, examination is directed to the sacrum and coccyx.

Examination

Inspection may show swelling or bruising or both over this area. Palpation will reveal a localized area of acute tenderness within the area of general pain.

X-Ray examination

The antero-posterior view may show gross deformity of the sacrum as part of fractures elsewhere in the pelvis. The lateral view of the sacrum and coccyx may show fracture usually around the sacro-coccygeal junction, with deformity and break in continuity, but most frequently no fracture is present.

Treatment

Fractures of the sacrum

Patients with comminuted or displaced fractures should be admitted to the orthopaedic wards for a few days for observation in case of visceral damage.

Localized fractures or contusions of the sacro-coccygeal junction

The pain from severe bruising of this area can be just as severe as that from a fracture. Therefore, whether the X-ray shows a fracture or not, treatment is required to relieve the pain. Only with fractures producing gross deformity is it necessary to attempt reduction; otherwise, the treatment of fracture or bruise is by thorough infiltration of the tender area with 1 per cent lignocaine. At the end of the infiltration, there should be no tenderness or deep palpation of the area. The patient should then be advised to use a soft cushion when sitting and to avoid constipation. With these precautions recovery can be expected within 2 to 3 weeks.

GROUP 4 — PAIN ON WALKING

A number of patients will attend complaining of pain in the hip or a limp, following a minor injury which occurred some days previously. These patients are frequently either old people or young children.

Elderly patients

Examination will reveal limitation of movement at the hip joint with pain at extremes of movement. Rarely, an impacted fracture of the neck of the femur may be the cause of symptoms, but in the vast majority osteo-arthrosis of the hip is present. If X-ray examination reveals a bony abnormality, the patient should be referred to the care of his general practitioner for treatment of a chronic degenerative condition or admitted to hospital when a fracture or malignancy is demonstrated.

Children

Because there are many causes of a limp in children, such as an infected blister on the heel with lymphadenitis in the groin, every child merits a full examination, even though this history of trauma may be insignificant. In these days one should never find an undiagnosed congenital dislocation

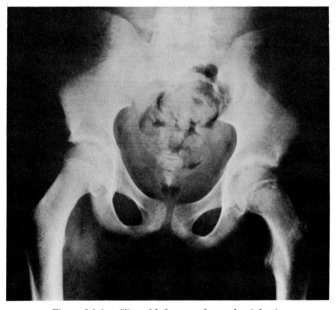

Figure 14.4.   Slipped left upper femoral epiphysis

of the hip as the cause of a limp, or rather a waddling gait, in a toddler, but if such a tragedy is discovered it requires immediate referral for orthopaedic treatment. At a slightly older age of 4 to 10 years, osteo-chondritis of the upper femoral epiphysis with flattening, and possibly later fragmentation of the epiphysis (Perthes disease) is an important but uncommon cause which requires orthopaedic treatment.

Acute or chronic microbial infections of the hip joints are also fortunately now rare in Great Britain. 'Transient synovitis', however, is a common condition. The physical signs of a synovitis of the hip are a painful joint with a reduced range of movement. A flexion deformity is the most characteristic single sign. To discover it the child should be lying flat on his back and the sound limb flexed to its fullest extent up to the abdominal wall. When a flexion deformity is present the thigh of the affected limb will be spontaneously raised off the couch and cannot be made to lie flat again. It is advisable to admit any child who exhibits such a sign for observation and possible further investigation. If physical and radiological examinations are both negative the mother can be reassured and asked to bring the child back if the symptoms have not completely disappeared in 4 to 5 days. A normal erythrocyte sedimentation rate is helpful in reaching the decision.

One other important orthopaedic condition which often presents at the A & E Department is that of slipped upper femoral epiphysis (*Figure 14.4*). This disorder more than any other illustrates the fact that disease in the hip may present as pain in the knee. Consequently any child between the ages of 9 and 14 years complaining of spontaneous onset of a vague pain around the knee should have his hips examined. Limitation of movement in the hip indicates the necessity for radiological examination and urgent orthopaedic advice should be sought for any patient who has asymmetrical upper femoral epiphyses.

15

Injuries to the Thigh and Knee

The knee joint is a gracious joint. If you take time to find out the precise details of the accident and pay the joint the compliment of a thorough physical examination, it will yield up most of its secrets and the diagnosis will become clear. Every injured knee joint must be examined in a comprehensive and systematic manner. To do this the patient must have his trousers removed or her skirt pulled up and tights removed and be lying on his/her back on a couch with good overhead illumination. The examination has four consecutive stages: look, feel, move and X-ray. By the time the third stage is completed the radiological findings of the fourth stage will often be predictable or, indeed, an X-ray examination may have become unnecessary.

HISTORY

There are 4 basic questions to ask:

1. How long is it since the injury occurred?
2. What was the exact nature of the injury?
3. How have the symptoms evolved since the accident happened?
4. Are there any other local or general medical factors which might be relevant?

How long?

Unless prevented by exceptional circumstances, a patient with a fracture or a serious injury to a ligament or tendon around the knee joint comes to hospital within 24 hours of the accident occurring. Patients who wait more than a day before seeking medical aid either have a mild effusion which is taking time to resolve, or they had previous pathology in or around the knee joint which has been aggravated or 'brought to light' by the injury.

What exactly happened?

A direct blow on the patella from a fall on the point of the knee, or crushing the knee against the dashboard of a car in a road traffic accident, will produce a fracture of the patella. In the car accident the force may also have been transmitted up to the hip joint producing a fracture or dislocation or both, so when the leg is injured in a car accident always examine the hip as well (*see Figure 14.3*).

A blow from the bumper of a car hitting the outside of a pedestrian's leg will produce an impacted, depressed fracture of the lateral condyle of the tibia.

A twisting injury, in which the foot remains fixed to the ground and the body swings round, is the classic method of producing a torn meniscus.

The elderly person who stumbles over a raised paving stone, falls to the ground and then cannot fully extend the knee, will have ruptured the quadriceps tendon.

What happened next?

Was it possible to continue working for a while or to continue playing after the accident occurred? Did the swelling come on immediately — probably haemarthrosis — or did it come on slowly over the next few hours — most likely a serous effusion.

Was it possible to extend the knee fully after the accident? Has there been 'locking' of the knee? This is a very useful item of information provided the patient fully understands what is meant. 'Surgical locking', implying a torn meniscus, means that the patient can extend the knee to a certain point and then no further. The loss of full extension may be only 15° but it is definite and consistent. The doctor must always be sure that a patient's description of 'locking' conforms with this definition.

Other relevant medical history

The child at puberty, especially an overweight boy, may have a traction apophysitis of the tibial apophysis (Osgood-Schlatter's disease). A patient with a bleeding diathesis may have a spontaneous haemarthrosis. Most common of all is the patient with osteoarthrosis of the knee joint. Such patients have managed fairly well until some relatively trivial injury aggravates their previously mild symptoms and makes them seek medical help.

PHYSICAL EXAMINATION

Look

Stand back and look at the knee in a good light, comparing it with the opposite knee. The swollen deformity from a fracture of femur or tibia may be obvious. Dislocation of the patella, most common in young women, presents as a rigid, painful knee with a lump on the lateral side. When the patella tendon is torn — a young person's injury — the patella lies higher than on the other side. When the quadriceps tendon is torn

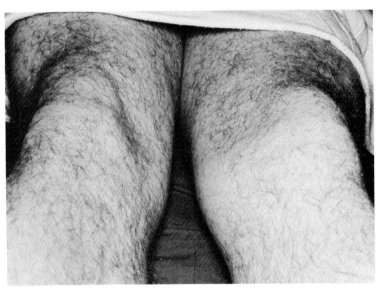

Figure 15.1.   This patient shows a normal para-patella fossa on the right but the left knee has a slight effusion and the fossa has filled out

— an old person's injury — there is a characteristic gap or hollow an inch above the patella. Dislocation of the knee — a rare but disastrous injury — presents with the leg no longer in line with the thigh and one's first concern must be for the circulation below the knee.

Fluid or inflammation in the bursae around the knee joint will be seen as localized swellings — pre-patella or infra-patella or behind the knee on the medial side — a semi-membranosus bursa. Effusion into the knee joint itself shows first of all by filling out the para-patella fossae — the hollows that normally lie on each side of the knee cap (*Figure 15.1*). Then the supra-patella bursa will fill and finally the whole joint may be bulging with a tense effusion of 100 ml or more.

Feel

First of all check the circulation in the limb, if necessary by palpation of the posterior tibial and dorsalis pedis arteries; then seek to localize the tenderness. A torn meniscus produces tenderness precisely along the joint line in the sulcus between femur and tibia on the appropriate side. A partially torn collateral ligament produces a more diffuse tenderness reaching up to the femoral condyle.

In the presence of a large effusion there will be a 'patella tap'. The patella is being held off the femoral condyles by the fluid in the joint; pressing on it depresses it a few millimetres until it impinges on the femur. A dislocated patella will be palpable on the lateral side of the joint. A fractured patella will be covered by bruising and oedema and it may be possible to elicit crepitus as bony fragments are palpated. A torn patella tendon results in a high riding patella with a hollow distal to it, and a ruptured quadriceps tendon leaves a soggy hollow just proximal to the patella.

Swellings limited to individual bursae will be palpable and the area will be warm and tender if there is active inflammation.

Localized hard lumps around the joint may be due to loose bodies, which will move as they are palpated; osteophytes which do not move; or, on the lateral aspect below the joint line, a cyst of the lateral cartilage. Small mobile loose bodies in the pre-patella bursa may be palpated; they give rise to pain on kneeling and require surgical removal.

Move

As with all joints, the movements are either active or passive. Examine the range of active movements first. Can the patient fully extend the knee? How far can he flex it compared with the opposite knee? Finally can he lift the heel off the couch without bending the knee — a test for the integrity of the extensor mechanism.

Passive movements are used to assess the integrity of the ligaments and the menisci. To examine the medial collateral ligament of the knee joint flex the knee $10-15°$, take hold of the ankle from the medial side with one hand, then place the other hand over the lateral aspect of the knee joint. Now apply a 'valgus strain' — trying to move the ankle away from the midline while holding the knee still with the other hand. One of 3 things will happen:

1. There will be no movement and the patient will not complain — the medial collateral ligament is intact.

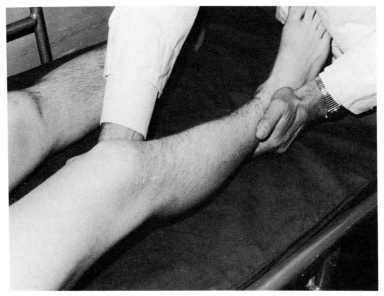

Figure 15.2.   Applying a valgus strain to the knee joint to test the integrity of the lateral collateral ligament

2. There will be little or no movement but the patient will complain of pain on the medial side of the knee joint — there is a partial tear of the medial collateral ligament.
3. There will be movement, but not necessarily much pain. When you relax the strain the leg will spring back into line and you will feel the impact as femoral and tibial condyles come back into contact. This is referred to as 'springing' of the joint — there is a complete tear of the medial collateral ligament. It may be accompanied by a dimple forming in the skin overlying the tear.

Now reverse the position of the hands and test the lateral collateral ligament (*Figure 15.2*).

Next, examine the cruciate ligaments. With the knee flexed to 45° take hold of the leg with both hands just below the knee and attempt to rock the tibia forwards and backwards. If the cruciates are slack there will be a few millimetres of movement. If they are torn there may be several centimetres of movement unless there is a large effusion which, by tightening the capsule, prevents the movement.

Finally, perform McMurray's manoeuvre to elicit the click of a torn cartilage. Stand beside the knee, place the upper hand over the front of the knee joint, fingers on one side, thumb on the other. Take hold of the dorsum of the foot with the other hand. Flex the knee as far as it will go, then rotate the tibia on the femur, first one way and extend the knee then, after re-applying flexion, rotate the tibia the other way and extend the knee. A click, heard or felt, during this manoeuvre, coupled with tenderness along the joint line indicates a torn meniscus. Unfortunately, within an hour or two of injury there may be such a large effusion in the joint that this manoeuvre is not possible. The effusion must be treated and the test applied when the swelling has subsided in about a week's time.

X-Ray

Antero-posterior and lateral views will show fractures or dislocations, changes due to osteo-arthrosis or other local pathology in the bones

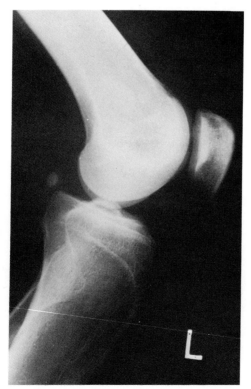

Figure 15.3.   A fabella is a sesamoid bone in the head of the gastrocnemius (not to be confused with a loose body)

around the joint. Loose bodies due to osteochondritis dissecans may be seen but to demonstrate the defect in the femoral condyle, from which they have come, a 'tunnel view' through the intercondylar notch is usually necessary. A fabella, a sesamoid bone in the lateral head of gastrocnemius (*Figure 15.3*) must not be confused with a loose body.

Careful scrutiny of the cortical line of each bone should reveal any fractures. The head and neck of the fibula should be included in the film and they merit special attention because of the close association of the lateral popliteal nerve with the neck of the fibula and the attachment of the lateral collateral ligament of the knee joint to the head of the fibula. Most fractures around the knee are so gross as to be obvious at first glance but a fracture of one of the tibial spines, to which the cruciate ligaments are attached, may be missed if the upper surface of the tibia is not examined carefully.

TREATMENT

If the circulation is impaired, steps to restore it by manipulation or open operation take precedence over all other local considerations.

Fractures of the femur

These are treated by the application of a Thomas splint. If the procedure is painful, we strongly recommend the use of entonox (50 per cent nitrous oxide and 50 per cent oxygen) to allow an approximate reduction of the fracture and the application of the splint. Check the circulation again after putting on the splint. The patient is then admitted to the orthopaedic ward.

Fractures of the upper end of tibia and fibula

These are usually treated with a long leg plaster of Paris cast but a severely depressed fracture of the lateral tibial condyle may require open reduction and internal fixation.

Dislocation of the knee

This should be reduced as quickly as possible using entonox or a general anaesthetic because of the risk to the circulation. The patient will then be admitted to the orthopaedic ward with his leg in a Thomas splint.

Dislocated patella

It may be possible to reduce the dislocation by pressure on the outer side of the patella. If this proves too painful, entonox will allow an easy reduction. A compression bandage should be applied, crutches prescribed, and the patient referred to the Fracture Clinic.

Fracture of the patella

If the patient can lift the heel off the couch with the knee extended, then the extensor aponeurosis must still be intact despite the fracture of the patella and an ankle-to-groin plaster of Paris cylinder should be applied and the patient referred to the Fracture Clinic. Otherwise the patient must be admitted to hospital for reconstruction or excision of the patella.

Tendinous and ligamentous tears

Partial tears of the collateral ligaments, if accompanied by a sizable effusion, should be treated by a Robert Jones compression bandage for 5 to 7 days, followed by a plaster of Paris cylinder when the swelling has subsided. If the effusion is small, at the time of the initial visit the plaster cylinder can be applied immediately and worn for 2 to 3 weeks. The complete tear should be referred to an orthopaedic surgeon with a view to surgical reconstruction. Tears of the patella tendon or the quadriceps tendon also require admission to hospital for surgical repair.

Torn meniscus

As already mentioned, it may be difficult to make this diagnosis at the initial visit because of the accompanying effusion. However, some patients come in considerable pain with the knee locked in about 60° of flexion. A general anaesthetic is required to allow manipulation to unlock the knee. A Robert Jones bandage is then applied and the patient referred for definitive surgery when the effusion has subsided.

Traction apophysitis (Osgood-Schlatter's disease)

Occasionally children, usually boys, between the ages of 10 and 15 years limp into the Emergency Department. They are found to have a swollen, tender area over the tibial tubercle and the insertion of quadriceps tendon. Usually a supporting bandage and instructions to avoid cycling and football are all that is required. For the more refractory causes a plaster of Paris cylinder for 1 to 2 months may be necessary.

Traumatic synovitis

The number of patients with this diagnosis will probably equal or surpass the total of all other patients with injuries around the knee joint. This is because the knee responds to any moderate trauma by forming a serous effusion in the joint. This is frequently seen in the knee which has early arthritic changes. The knee is generally tender and movements are restricted. Occasionally the effusion is so large that the knee is bulging and the patient is in considerable pain. This situation justifies aspiration of the joint. After full surgical preparation, with an aseptic technique, fluid is aspirated through a needle introduced on the lateral aspect of the joint under the upper half of the patella. The aspirate may contain globules of fat, indicating that there is a fracture involving the knee joint, or it may contain blood – a haemarthrosis.

After the aspiration, or immediately if aspiration is not necessary, the knee joint must be immobilized. Traditionally this has been done by applying a Robert Jones bandage. This consists of a layer of cotton wool bandaged in place by a flannel bandage, then a second layer of wool and bandage, then a third layer! This bulky dressing, it is claimed, provides both rest for the knee joint by preventing flexion, and compression on the joint to discourage the effusion from recurring. Critics of the treatment maintain that pressure sufficient to stop the effusion re-forming must also impair the circulation in the leg generally and they prefer to use a padded plaster of Paris cylinder.

Tone in the quadriceps muscle should be maintained by teaching the patient to do 'static exercises', that is tightening and relaxing the muscle within the bandage or plaster cast for, say, 5 minutes every 3 hours. Cast or bandage should be removed after a week and replaced with an elasticated support, such as Tubigrip, and the patient can start walking, with the aid of crutches or a stick if necessary. If they have not kept up the tone in the quadriceps muscle the patients may complain of the knee 'giving way' as they walk. This complaint, together with pain and a chronic effusion, will only disappear when muscle power returns to normal. The wearing of platform shoes significantly retards or prevents recovery.

Bursitis

Either the pre-patellar or the infra-patellar bursa may become swollen or inflamed. Usually this follows repetitive minor trauma and it may be complicated by bacterial infection. Incision is not recommended as the surgical wound is often slow to heal. Aspiration will relieve the pain and give a sample of fluid for bacteriological study. A compression bandage, rest, and if necessary antibiotic therapy should produce a cure within a week to 10 days. The patient must then take care to protect the knee or avoid the trauma which precipitated the acute episode.

Myositis ossificans

Although this condition may develop following trauma around the elbow joint it is seen most frequently in the thigh. The usual story is of a blow on the thigh during a football game. After the game the thigh becomes increasingly painful and flexion of the joint aggraves the pain. Over the

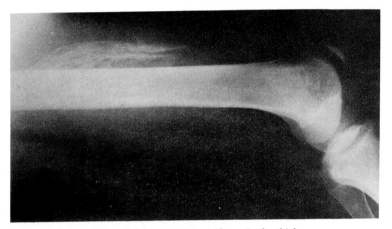

Figure 15.4.   Myositis ossificans in the thigh

next few days a firm swelling, some 10–15 cm in diameter, develops in the thigh. Massage or exercises only serve to aggravate the symptoms. The patient comes to the Accident Department complaining of the painful swelling and a range of flexion of less than 90°. The typical history with these findings on physical examination gives the clinical diagnosis of myositis ossificans. The substantive diagnosis is made by X-ray examination (*Figure 15.4*). This radiological evidence, an area of hazy calcification lying anterior to the femoral shaft, is not seen for at least 10 days after the injury and may not appear for 6 weeks. Treatment, therefore, should be started on the clinical diagnosis alone and X-rays taken at weekly intervals to check for the appearance of a calcified shadow and then to document its progress.

Treatment consists of stopping all massage or exercises and putting the thigh at rest by applying a plaster of Paris cylinder. This immobilization should continue for 6 weeks or until all local tenderness in the thigh has gone, whichever is the longer. Thereafter, gradual knee exercises can be started under physiotherapy supervision. Any recurrence of pain in the thigh at this time indicates the need for a further 3 weeks' immobilization. By this time the X-ray appearance may show a dense, bone-like shadow in the thigh, but once the edges of the shadow are smooth and well defined the condition will not grow any further and the patient can hope to return to a full range of sporting activity.

16

Injuries to the Leg and Ankle

These common injuries will be described under 3 headings:

1. Injuries to bones.
2. Injuries to muscles.
3. Injuries to tendons and ligaments.

So far as injuries to the bones are concerned, only the broad principles will be mentioned and the reader is recommended to consult a standard textbook on fracture management for the details of treatment (e.g. *Closed Treatment of Common Fractures,* Charnley, J., Churchill Livingstone, 1976; *System of Orthopaedics and Fractures,* Apley, A. G., Butterworths 1977.)

FRACTURES

All open fractures must be admitted to hospital under the care of an orthopaedic surgeon. In the Emergency Department the doctor must check the circulation distal to the fracture, apply a temporary sterile dressing, if necessary give an analgesic injection and apply temporary splintage. It is important to make sure that there is no central trauma to head, thorax or abdomen, which could threaten life, before turning all one's attention to the peripheral injury. Also, remember that the limb may be injured at more than one level. Fractures or dislocations of the hip can easily be overlooked because of a fracture of the leg which is more obvious and more painful.

Closed fractures (*Figure 16.1*) will be treated initially either by the emergency doctor or by the orthopaedic staff according to local arrangements and depending on the severity of the injury. Fractures of the tibia and fibula, if displaced, will be reduced under a general anaesthetic and then, as with undisplaced fractures, immobilized in an above-knee plaster of Paris cast. Only if the fracture affects one malleolus only, and the fracture line is distal to the level of the main tibio-talar articular surface, should a below-knee plaster cast be used.

162

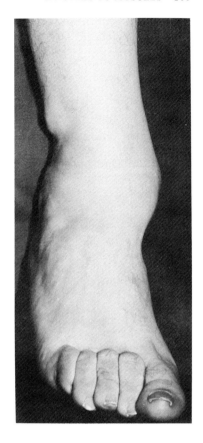

Figure 16.1. Bimalleolar fracture with subluxation of the ankle joint

All these plaster of Paris casts must be padded, and the patient must not bear weight on them for at least the first 24 hours. The circulation in the toes must be checked after 24 hours, the patient having been instructed to seek medical advice earlier if the toes become swollen or blue.

INJURIES TO MUSCLES

Anterior compartment syndrome

This patient complains of pain down the front of the leg aggravated by walking or running. The syndrome is seen most frequently in people who have made an extraordinary muscular effort or in an athlete who has just started training. Presumably there has been a partial muscle tear of the dorsiflexor muscles with bleeding in the closely confined compartment between tibia and fibula. Resting the leg as much as possible and Diapulse therapy to dissipate the oedema will relieve the symptoms.

Injury to the calf muscles

Following a sudden muscular effort, such as running to catch a bus, a patient complains of pain in the calf. Palpation will reveal a localized area of tenderness due to rupture of some of the fibres of gastrocnemius muscle. Treatment is to have a 1–1.5 cm raise on the heel of the shoe of the affected leg for a couple of weeks. Bandaging, especially in female patients taking the contraceptive pill, is not recommended because of the risk of local thrombosis and possible embolism.

INJURIES TO TENDONS AND LIGAMENTS

Ruptured Achilles tendon

This condition is seen in middle-aged people, especially if they are over-weight. A common cause is the so-called 'keep-fit' class. A complete tear is such a dramatic event that the patients look round to see who has hit them. Then, finding that they can no longer rise onto their toes but only shuffle along flat-footed, they usually make the diagnosis themselves. Treatment is by surgical repair.

A partial tear of the tendon presents as a painful swelling behind and above the heel, but without the characteristic gap that occurs when the tendon is completely torn. The patient can still plantar flex the foot against resistance, but it is painful to do so. Treatment is to apply a below-knee plaster of Paris cast with the ankle in equinus to rest the tendon. This is the only situation in which the foot should be immobilized in plantar flexion. The patient is then referred to an orthopaedic surgeon for subsequent management.

The recent surge of enthusiasm for 'jogging', particularly amongst middle-aged men, many of whom are seeking rehabilitation after a coronary thrombosis, has resulted in an increase in the number of patients with partial tears and strains of the calf muscles or tendons.

Sprained ankle

This extremely common condition falls into 3 catagories; the minor injury, the severe, and a broad intermediate group.

Minor injury

Most people who sustain a minor sprain look after it themselves but a few come to hospital. They walk in with little or no limp and the swelling and tenderness are minimal. They need reassurance, advice and perhaps a crêpe bandage.

Severe injury

These are patients in whom the stability of the ankle joint is at risk or disrupted. Their lesion is extremely painful, they cannot bear weight on the foot, there is gross swelling and tenderness. An X-ray of the ankle may show fractures of medial or lateral malleoli or both, the fracture line being sufficiently high in the malleolus to remove one of the buttresses of the ankle mortice. If no bony injury is shown on X-ray, films taken with the foot stressed into maximum inversion, then maximum eversion will show if there is movement of the talus within the ankle mortice due to complete rupture of medial or lateral ligaments (*Figure 16.2*). To perform this investigation adequately in the acute stage may require the use of entonox or intravenous analgesia (e.g. 10 mg Diazepam). If the sprain, or rupture, involves the medial, deltoid ligament surgical repair is recommended. If only the lateral ligament is involved, opinions vary as to whether surgical repair or plaster of Paris immobilization is indicated in this situation. The emergency doctor should consult his orthopaedic colleague.

Moderate injury

This group of patients are often incapacitated by their injury, even though the integrity of the ankle joint is not in doubt. They provide a substantial part of the work of the A & E Department. An inversion injury, producing a sprain or partial tear of the lateral ligament of the ankle is the most common. Because the medial ligament is stronger than the lateral it is not sprained so easily but, when it is, it implies that there has been a considerable amount of force involved in the accident and an X-ray examination is advisable.

The lateral ligament has its origin at the lower end of the fibula, or lateral malleolus and it fans out with 3 distinct bands. The talo-fibular ligament is sprained when the inversion injury occurs with the ankle fully plantar flexed as in the take-off position when running. The pain, swelling and tenderness are then below and anterior to the lateral malleolus. Pain and swelling immediately below the lateral malleolus

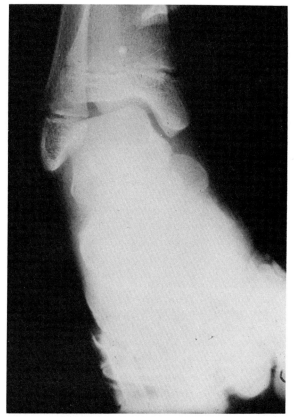

*Figure 16.2.   A stress film of the ankle showing movement
of the talus within the mortice. The patient has a tear of the
lateral ligament but no bony injury*

implies that the fibulo-cuboid ligament has been sprained, which occurs
when the inversion injury takes place with the foot in the neutral
position. The fibulo-calcaneal ligament is rarely torn in isolation.

The tip of either malleolus may be fractured off in this type of injury.
If there was an element of rotation in the force applied to the ankle, the
lateral malleolus may be fractured obliquely. This fracture line is often
invisible on the antero-posterior film, and will only be seen following
careful scrutiny of the lateral film because the medial malleolus and
talus are in the same line of projection.

The same type of inversion injury may produce a fracture of the base
of the fifth metatarsal due to the pull of peroneus brevis tendon in its

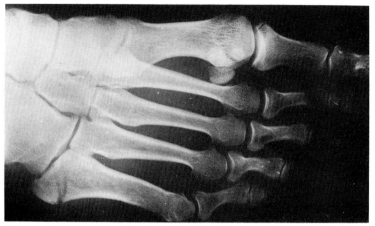

Figure 16.3.   Fracture of the base of the fifth metatarsal. This commonly occurs as part of a 'sprained ankle' injury

attempt to take the whole weight of the body (*Figure 16.3*). On palpation of these bony points — the malleolus and the base of the fifth metatarsal — it may be possible to decide that there is no bony injury present. If one can state this with confidence, then no X-ray is necessary. If there is any doubt at all, take an X-ray of the ankle to show the malleoli, and an X-ray of the foot to show the fifth metatarsal. Reviewing these patients has shown us that the incidence of fractures associated with sprained ankles is 4 times greater in patients over 50 years of age than in younger patients.

If a fracture is demonstrated on X-ray then a below-knee plaster of Paris cast is applied and the patient referred to the Fracture Clinic.

If there is no fracture, the intensity with which the lesion is treated depends on the urgency with which the patient wishes to return to full activity. If there is no great urgency then adhesive strapping is applied from toes to calf. The patient is advised to rest the ankle for 24 to 48 hours and then gradually to resume walking. After a week to 10 days when the strapping is removed, the symptoms are usually greatly improved. A crêpe bandage or tubigauze may be required for a further week.

For the patient for whom 2 weeks is too long a period of reduced activity, physiotherapy can speed recovery. Ultrasound or Diapulse therapy will disperse the oedema and thereby reduce the pain. If this is followed by supportive bandaging and supervised walking exercises, treatment on 3 successive days will relieve most of the symptoms. A double blind trial using Diapulse therapy showed that on average 80 per cent of symptoms were relived after 3 days of treatment (Wilson, D. H., 1971, *Br. med. J.* 2, 269).

17

Injuries to the Foot

Patients coming to the Accident and Emergency Department with foot problems fall into 1 of 2 groups:

1. Those who have sustained a specific, recent injury.
2. Those with pain in the foot of recent onset, whose symptoms are attributed to some recent imprecise minor injury.

Physical examination of a recently injured foot will elicit pain and swelling, but it is not usually possible to make a definite diagnosis without an X-ray examination. Because patients wish to walk on their feet, that is to transmit their whole body weight through each foot in turn, it is important to know if the bony structures are intact and this necessitates a radiological examination. Emergency management of the more common injuries of the foot are as described below.

GROUP 1 − A RECENT SPECIFIC INJURY

Fractures of the calcaneum

This fracture results from a fall from a height onto the heels. The patient is carried into hospital with a painful swollen heel. It is essential to remember that the force of the fall may well have been transmitted up the leg to the hip and spine producing fractures at either or both of these levels − even though the patient does not immediately complain of them.

If the fracture involves the subtaloid joint and there is extensive swelling, the patient should be admitted to hospital for elevation of the foot and early exercises, in order to minimize, so far as possible, the long-term complications of stiffness and pain in the foot.

For fractures not involving the talo-calcaneal joint a well padded below-knee plaster of Paris cast or a wool and crêpe dressing is applied and the patient referred to the Fracture Clinic. Patients with fractures of both os calces may require admission to hospital for social reasons.

Fracture of the talus

This fortunately rare injury should always receive early expert ortho-paedic treatment because of:

1. The risks of necrosis of the skin if there is a dislocation associated with the fracture.
2. Avascular necrosis of the head of the talus.
3. A permanently painful stiff foot.

Mid-tarsal dislocation

This injury produces a very painful swollen foot. A junior doctor exam-ining the X-ray may fail to appreciate the seriousness of the injury because there is no fracture. Examining the radiological appearance of each individual bone is necessary but one must also study the relation-ship of each bone with its neighbours. In this condition the proximal articular surface of the navicular is no longer articulating with the head of the talus, and a reduction under anaesthetic is required. The sooner the manipulation is attempted, the easier it is; delay allows oedema to develop and makes the reduction more difficult. Following the reduction a well padded plaster cast is applied and the patient instructed to elevate the foot – and sleep with it on a pillow for the next 48 hours. Admis-sion to hospital may be necessary after the reduction in order to supervise the circulation. A bipartite or accessory navicular bone must not be mis-diagnosed as a fracture of the navicular; it is recognizable by its smooth, rounded, clearly defined edges.

Fractures of the metatarsals

Fracture of the base of the fifth metatarsal is discussed in Chapter 16 under 'Sprained ankles'. Fractures of the shafts of the metatarsals do not usually need any manipulation; a padded below-knee plaster of Paris cast is the appropriate treatment.

Fractures of the necks of the metatarsals often occur in the guise of a 'March fracture'. After a long hike in heavy footwear the patient complains of pain and tenderness in the region of the necks of the second or third metatarsals. At this stage an X-ray may fail to show a fracture. Elastoplast strapping from toes to calf will give sufficient support. If the symptoms are still present after 2 weeks a second X-ray may show bone resorption at the site of the fracture with a small amount of callus around it. This, a 'March fracture', is well on the way to being healed and only symptomatic treatment is necessary.

170

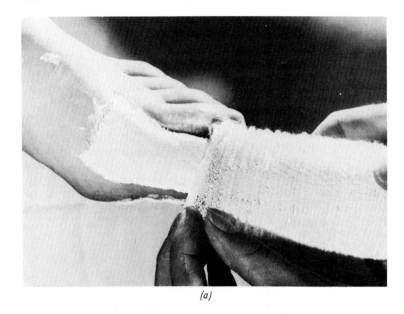

(a)

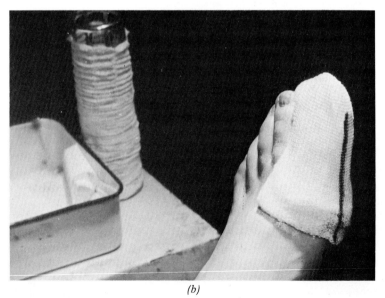

(b)

Figure 17.1.   (a) Applying a plaster of Paris slab to the dorsal surface of a fractured hallux. (b) The edge of the plaster of Paris is indicated by a line on the tubigauze. Cutting along this line makes removal of the splint easy and painless

Fracture of the toes

The hallux

Crushing injuries of the big toe are very common in areas of heavy industry. Protective footwear with steel toe caps should make the injury a rarity — but this has yet to happen. Manipulation of the fractured phalanges is rarely necessary and treatment is directed towards protecting the toe until the tenderness disappears and healing is well advanced. This is done by applying a plaster of Paris slab or a collodion splint over the toe and, if necessary, applying a pad of orthopaedic felt under the heads of the metatarsals. With this treatment most patients can return to work within a couple of weeks (*Figure 17.1*).

The smaller toes

Displacement requiring manipulation is rare. Simple immobilization by strapping the injured toe to its uninjured neighbour for 1 to 2 weeks is all that is necessary (*Figure 17.2*). Painting gentian violet 1:200 between toes before applying the strapping discourages an exacerbation of the all too common 'athlete's foot'.

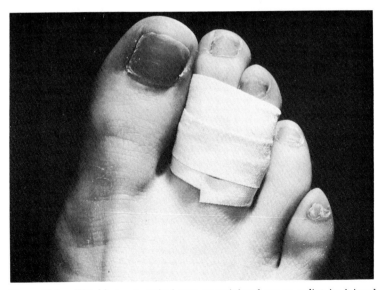

Figure 17.2.   'Neighbour strapping' uses an uninjured toe to splint its injured neighbour

The treatment of the bruised smaller toe without a fracture is exactly the same and it is doubtful, therefore, if X-ray examination of an injured smaller toe is necessary.

Injured feet in small children

The young child is not able to localize accurately a pain in the leg. He limps in, or is carried in, and complains of a pain in the foot. It is wise to examine the leg as well as the foot, because an undisplaced spiral fracture of the tibia may well present in this way.

GROUP 2 – NO RECENT SPECIFIC INJURY

'Osteochondritis'

In children and adolescents, avascular necrosis of the navicular bone (Kohler's disease), or a similar osteochondritis of the heads of the second or third metatarsals (Freiberg's disease) – this latter condition being more common in young adults – may produce pain in the foot. On X-ray the navicular looks dense and small, the metatarsal heads are broad and flat with a thickened neck. The symptoms usually respond to supportive bandaging. Only occasionally is it necessary to excise the metatarsal head in Freiberg's disease.

Metatarsalgia

Pain across the metatarsal joints is a common condition in older people probably due to being overweight and having poor tone in the intrinsic muscles of the foot. 'Emergency treatment', if this is ever necessary, consists of applying a metatarsal pad under the metatarsal heads and referring the patient for an orthopaedic opinion.

Hallux rigidus

While out walking, an otherwise healthy patient, experiences a sudden pain in the first metatarso-phalangeal joint. The pain may last a few minutes or a few hours. On examination the joint is stiff, tender and painful especially on dorsi flexion. In younger patients there will be no radiological abnormality but as the years pass osteo-arthritic changes become increasingly evident. Treatment in the first instance is by applying a metatarsal pad for a week or so. The patient must make sure that his shoes are not too tight and crowding his toes.

Gout

The middle-aged or elderly male patient who wakes with a painful tender first metatarso-phalangeal joint almost certainly has gout. While awaiting the results of a serum uric acid estimation, a therapeutic trial of 200 mg phenylbutazone 3 times a day, will support the diagnosis by bringing rapid relief.

In-growing toe nails

This condition is very common in young men who wear tight socks and shoes and who forget to wash their feet regularly. Incorrect cutting of the toe nails by delving down with the scissors into the grooves at each side of the nail also promotes the complaint. Toe nails should be cut square across the ends. Treatment, if the toe is infected, is usually by removal of the nail under a digital block, and the application of a medicated tulle dressing. If the condition recurs a definitive 'cure' is achieved by radical removal of the nail and nail bed — Zadik's operation. A less radical procedure, which is gaining popularity, is the chiropody treatment of a wedge re-section of the nail and cauterization of the appropriate section of the nail bed with 80 per cent phenol so that the offending lateral border of the nail does not grow again.

18

The Treatment of Wounds

INTRODUCTION

The treatment of wounds is one of the most important parts of the work of an Accident and Emergency Department. The surgeon in charge and the nursing officer must establish a policy and set up a routine which all the staff should follow. The results of this work must be constantly under review so that improvements will come from agreed modifications of the policy. Individual, haphazard variations in the routine usually result in a lowering of the standard of work. The following 9 steps form a pattern which should be followed for all wounds. The department should be designed, equipped and staffed so that each step can be taken expeditiously and efficiently.

1. Assessment of the wound.
2. Preparation of the wound area.
3. Anaesthesia.
4. Suturing.
5. Dressing of the wound after suture.
6. Tetanus prevention.
7. Recording of the wound and details of the treatment.
8. Removal of sutures in the Dressing Clinic.
9. Rehabilitation.

The remainder of this chapter is a description of each of these steps in turn, with details of technique where appropriate.

ASSESSMENT OF THE WOUND

All wounds should be inspected with the patient screened from general view. A friend or relative should only be present if the age or mental state of the patient makes it necessary. Normally, other people do not wish to see bleeding wounds exposed to their gaze. The patient should at least be sitting down. When the wound is severe, involves the lower limb, or is causing undue distress, the patient should be lying down on a couch in a cubicle.

While the nurse removes the First Aid dressing, the doctor can take a brief history. This must elicit the cause, time and circumstance of the accident, and hence the possibility of fractures or injuries to other parts of the body and also of local complications such as the possible presence of foreign bodies, grease or oil or other contaminants.

Patients with major wounds or wounds which require the skill of a specialist surgeon will be admitted to the appropriate ward. Gun-shot wounds and stab wounds of the thorax or abdomen should also be admitted for a full surgical exploration. The management of hand injuries is described in Chapter 13.

The patient should be asked about his previous immunization against tetanus and sensitivity to any antibiotics which may be used.

At this time the doctor should write down the history, a description of the wound — for which a simple sketch is often helpful — and instructions for the patient's management. This will include, if necessary, X-ray for foreign bodies or associated fractures, preliminary preparation of the wound area and the type of anaesthesia to be used during suturing.

PREPARATION OF THE WOUND AREA

In the majority of wounds, the cleaning of the skin around the wound area will be done on the operating table immediately before suture. In a proportion of hand injuries in particular, however, the surrounding skin may be thickly coated with oil and grease or other dirt, and will create a problem for cleaning in the theatre. In these circumstances it is recommended that a proprietory hand cleanser, such as 'Swarfega' be used. The patient can do the cleaning himself and then be given a sterile, soft nail brush and a sterile bowl containing 1 per cent cetrimide to complete the cleaning of the skin. Since grease may contain anaerobic organisms, especially *Clostridium tetanii*, or, if left in the wound, may produce a painful granuloma, it is particularly important to remove it from the wound. Some crushed fingers are too painful for thorough cleaning until they have been numbed by a local anaesthetic digital nerve block. It is always wise to re-assess the wound after the preliminary cleaning and the necessity for a skin graft may be reconsidered. Hot tar, as used in road works, can be removed either by a proprietory hand cleanser or by olive oil followed by cetrimide toilet. Hot bitumen, as used in roofing, can be left on the skin unless it involves the eyes, mouth or flexion creases. Within 10 days the bitumen will fall off and the skin will have healed beneath it. Abrasions with dirt deeply ingrained require scrubbing with cetrimide and a sterile brush under an anaesthetic, otherwise the dirt will produce permanent tattooing.

ANAESTHESIA

The majority of wounds sutured in the A & E Department can, and should, be sutured under local anaesthetic. One per cent lignocaine without adrenaline can be infiltrated directly into the wound. A short, straight, clean incised wound, requiring only one stitch, may be closed by a skilful operator without an anaesthetic, but any wound which requires 2 or more sutures justifies local anaesthesia. Children may be helped by oral pre-operative sedation [e.g. 2.5 mg/kg Vallergan, or 2 mg (1–3 year-olds) or 4 mg (4–7 year-olds) of Valium] and the assistance of a co-operative, stoical parent; but extensive suturing, especially in children who are too young or too afraid to co-operate, requires general anaesthesia. In some wounds of the fingers, a digital nerve block at the base of the finger may be of more use than direct infiltration of local anaesthetic into the wound. In areas of tight tissue tension, where local anaesthetic injection is difficult and painful, mixing an ampoule or hyalase with 10 ml of 1 per cent lignocaine will facilitate the injection, but will of course shorten the duration of the anaesthesia.

SUTURING THE WOUND

Suturing a wound must be done as a 'sterile' procedure with the patient comfortably positioned and the area of the wound well illuminated. The operator must then observe the following basic principles:

1. Thoroughly clean the wound with gauze soaked in 1 per cent cetrimide.
2. Remove all dirt, foreign bodies or dead tissue.
3. Stop any continuing bleeding with a deep stitch or ligature.
4. Bring the remaining tissue into precise apposition using, if necessary, deep absorbable sutures before closing the skin edges in careful alignment.
5. Handle the tissues gently to avoid inflicting further trauma.
6. Tie the sutures firmly to avoid leaving dead space but do not strangle the tissue within the suture − it must have a blood supply in order to heal.
7. Do not suture the wound under tension.
8. When closing the skin, start in the middle of the wound or at jagged corners which will give precise locations on each margin of the wound. This will divide the wound into a number of straight segments which are then halved by each subsequent suture.
9. Remember that skin is living tissue and the wound edges will grow together, provided they have not been inverted, everted or

strangled by the sutures. The purpose of the sutures is to bring the skin edges together in precise apposition to facilitate this biological process of wound-healing. The suture of themselves cannot impart any strength to the wound.

10. Choice of suture material and size. For deep sutures the choice lies between, in order of preference: collagen, synthetic absorbable suture material, or catgut. For skin sutures an atraumatic needle should be used of a size appropriate to the wound. Monofilament nylon sutures are recommended for facial wounds because they will be removed after only 3 days. The same material is indicated for leg wounds, as the sutures should remain *in situ* for 2 weeks. For other wounds, and particularly for children, collagen sutures are preferred because the deep part will dissolve in 10 to 14 days and the exposed part will brush off when the dressing is removed. The suture size varies: 3/0 for a wound on the trunk or leg; 4/0 for an adult upper limb or scalp; 5/0 for a child's upper limb or an adult face; 6/0 for a child's face.

Special wounds

Treatment of wounds of the scalp is described in Chapter 4, wounds of the face and mouth in Chapter 5, and wounds of the hand in Chapter 13.

Deep abrasions

These are caused in 2 ways. In a road accident the patient slides along the road surface, the superficial skin is abraded and road dirt is embedded in the wound. Under general anaesthesia all dirt must be scrubbed out of the wound with a firm, sterile brush. Loose tags of superficial skin should be cut off. If the dermis is intact, the wound will re-epithelialize with minimal or no scarring. The second type of deep abrasion is potentially more serious. It occurs when a hand or forearm is trapped between moving rollers in an old wringing machine or an industrial accident. The skin may still be intact but the shearing force of the rollers, having torn the capillaries beneath the skin, will result in necrosis and sloughing. At the initial examination, if there is no capillary flush in response to pressure on the skin, the patient should be referred to a plastic surgeon with a view to excision and skin grafting.

Wounds of the shin

The circulation on the front of the leg is often very poor and wounds are slow to heal. Problems arise most frequently in elderly female patients who lacerate their shin on stairs, the platform of a bus, a shop

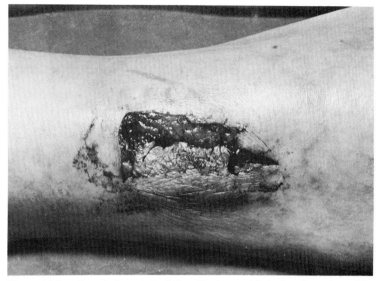

Figure 18.1.   A typical wound of the shin in an elderly female patient. After wound toilet and the application of sterile strips this wound was heeled in 12 days

display stand or similar objects. The injuries often produce a triangular wound with a flap or skin hanging loose at the base. If the length of the flap is more than half the length of its attached base, then necrosis around the edges of the flap is likely. In treating the wound, all loose or damaged fat should be gently cut away. The flap should then be loosely sutured in place, or the edges gently approximated by applying sterile adhesive strips, covering as much of the wound as is possible without applying any tension. This will often result in an area of the wound remaining uncovered. As the oedema subsides and the wound heals this exposed area will diminish in size, and only rarely is a secondary skin graft necessary (*Figure 18.1*). Conversely, if at the initial operation the flap is pulled tight by sutures so as to close the whole wound, it probably will slough and a much more extensive grafting procedure will be necessary. After the initial operation a non-adhesive, sterile dressing and a firm supporting bandage should be applied. The patient should be advised to reduce his daily activities, but not to stay in bed. When sitting, he should rest the leg on a stool or put it up on a settee or couch. The wound may be re-dressed after 1 week but the sutures should remain for 2 weeks, following which ultra-violet light therapy is useful to stimulate the closure of any part of the wound which remains unhealed. If the healing process fails to progress, the patient's general health and state of nutrition should be examined and further advice sought.

DRESSING OF THE WOUND AFTER SUTURE

Dressings are traditional and have a cosmetic value but their real purpose is to protect the wound from further trauma and to rest the part while the wound heals. If the skin is not completely closed, a non-adhesive tulle should be applied to prevent the main dressing sticking to the wound. No dressing should be as tight as to impair the circulation or produce oedema distal to the wound and it is important to ensure that this is so before the patient leaves the department. Adhesive strapping may be used to secure a dressing and so ensure that it has not dropped off by the time the patient reaches home; but in using it care must be taken not to produce a tourniquet effect and it should never be used so liberally as to enclose completely the dressing, since this invites infection due to retained perspiration. A triangular sling may be a useful additional item of dressing to remind the patient to rest an injury of the hand or forearm and to persuade other people to treat him gently for the next few days. A water permeable plastic dressing from an aerosol spray, is ideal for areas such as the face and scalp which will not be covered by clothing and are unlikely to be subjected to further trauma.

TETANUS PREVENTION AND THE USE OF ANTIBIOTICS

Tetanus still exists and is a constant threat following any open wound. A review of patients treated in the Tetanus Unit at the Leeds General Infirmary (Atrakchi, S. A. and Wilson, D. H., 1977, *Br. med. J.,* 1, 179) showed that sportsmen using muddy playing fields and people engaged in gardening or agricultural work, are particularly at risk. Tetanus also developed in two patients with chronic varicose ulcers and in several other patients who had only sustained apparently benign minor injuries.

In recent years tetanus immunization has been combined with dipthera and petussis in a triple vaccine. Anxiety over the occasional complications from the petussis element in the vaccination has resulted in the incidence of childhood immunization falling from 75 per cent to approximately 50 per cent, so half the children in Britain are now no longer protected against tetanus. The seriousness of this regrettable trend is partially masked by the fact that human tetanus immunoglobulin is now readily available; it is an expensive product which gives passive immunization lasting about 4 weeks. It is far safer and much more reliable than the equine anti-tetanus serum (commonly referred to as ATS). There is now no place for equine ATS in either tetanus prevention or treatment in Britain.

Active tetanus immunization should be prescribed for all non-immune patients who attend the A & E Department for treatment of any wound.

It consists of a course of 3 intramuscular injections of 0.5 ml of adsorbed tetanus toxoid given: one at the first visit, the second after 6 weeks, and the third after 6 months. This gives immunity for 10 years and a booster dose (again 0.5 ml) should be given at or before the expiry of the 10-year period.

When there are indications for giving passive immunization with human tetanus immunoglobulin, a dose of 250 units in 1 ml is given by intramuscular injection. Though extremely rare, an anaphylactic reaction may occur following this injection, and facilities for resuscitation should be available when the injection is given.

In every A & E Department there must be a firmly established routine for tetanus prevention. Smith, Laurence and Evans (Smith, J. W. G., Laurence, D. R. and Evans, D. G., 1975, *Br. med. J.,* 3, 453) proposed the following programme which is now widely accepted:

1. All wounds receive surgical toilet (this is the most important single aspect of the treatment programme).
2. Then they divide patients into 4 categories:
   A. Has had a complete course of toxoid or a booster dose within the past 5 years.
   B. Has had a complete course of toxoid or a booster dose more than 5 and less than 10 years ago.
   C. Has had a complete course of toxoid or a booster dose more than 10 years ago.
   D. Has not had a complete course of toxoid, or immunity status is unknown.
3. For patients with clean wounds (less than 6 hours old, non-penetrating and negligible tissue damage):
   Category A — nothing more required after surgical treatment of the wound.
   Categories B and C — booster dose of toxoid.
   Category D — complete course of toxoid.
4. For patients with dirty wounds (contaminated, infected, penetrating, more than 6 hours old or with extensive tissue damage.):
   Category A — nothing more required after surgical treatment of the wound so far as tetanus protection is concerned.
   Category B — booster dose of toxoid.
   Category C — booster dose of toxoid + human tetanus immunoglobulin.
   Category D — complete course of tetanus toxoid + human tetanus immunoglobulin.

Note: When both toxoid and immunoglobulin are indicated, they can be given at the same time but into different limbs.

RECORDING OF THE WOUND AND DETAILS OF THE TREATMENT

The patient's record card will already contain notes on the time, cause and circumstances of the accident. Precise details of the wound or wounds should now be added and again a sketch may be useful to indicate the site and extent of the injuries. The number of sutures and

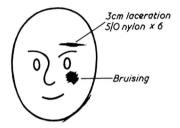

3cm laceration
S/O nylon x 6

Bruising

Figure 18.2.   A simple diagram is often better than words for describing injuries and their treatment

the suture material should be recorded and the presence or absence of other injuries noted (*Figure 18.2*). Injections must be recorded, especially tetanus prophylaxis, and the nurse who gives the injection should initial the card. Any prescription given to the patient must also be noted in detail on the record card. It is essential to complete the record card before proceeding to examine or treat another patient.

REMOVAL OF SUTURES IN THE DRESSING CLINIC

The introduction of collagen sutures which dissolve and drop off in 10 to 14 days has obviated much of the tedious and painful work of removing skin sutures. This is proving particularly valuable in treating children and patients with hand injuries. However, this does not excuse the surgeon from following up his patients and ensuring that the wounds are well healed. In facial wounds where the sutures will be removed in 3 days, and in leg wounds where the sutures are intended to remain *in situ* for 2 weeks, monofilament nylon sutures are still preferred and these must be removed in the Dressing Clinic.

When patients leave the department after the initial treatment, they should be told to return to any subsequent Dressing Clinic if they are worried; otherwise they should attend after the appropriate number of days according to the site of their injury. Changing the dressing and inspecting the wound before this is meddlesome and should be avoided if possible.

The following figures are given as a guide to the number of days after operation when the wound should be examined and non-absorbable sutures removed if the anticipated degree of healing has occurred:

Face, head and neck   3 days.
Arm and hand   7 days.
Trunk and lower limb   10–14 days.

REHABILITATION

After the wound has been inspected and non-absorbable sutures removed, the majority of patients can be discharged from the department and return to their normal activities. However, some patients with moderately

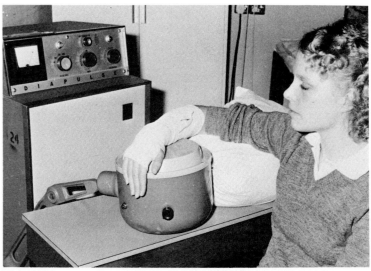

Figure 18.3.   Diapulse treatment given to reduce the pain, swelling and stiffness in an injured wrist

severe injuries of the wrist or hand may require a short period of rehabilitation before being able to return to work. In the field of electro-therapy, Diapulse treatment is proving useful in dispersing oedema and thereby reducing pain and stiffness, and this can be given through the dressing from the day of injury (*Figure 18.3*). Once the dressing is removed, wax therapy and hand exercises are helpful, and for some patients occupational therapy is indicated to enable them to regain skill and confidence in the use of their hands (*see Figure 13.6*). Close liaison between the surgeon and the staff of the rehabilitation department will produce excellent results.

19

The Treatment of Burns and Scalds

INTRODUCTION

A scald is caused by hot liquids; a burn may be caused by dry heat, electricity, friction, chemicals or radioactivity. Any of these causes may produce either a 'partial thickness' lesion, where only the epidermis and the superficial part of the dermis is destroyed, or they may produce a 'full thickness' burn in which the lesion extends through the dermis to the subcutaneous tissue. In the partial thickness burn the uninjured, deeper layer of the dermis retains the ability to re-epithelialize the affected area, but in the full thickness burn healing will be by scar

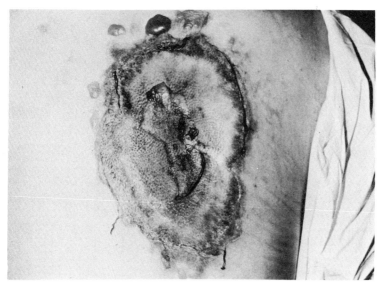

Figure 19.1.   Deep burn of the back, caused by a hot-water bottle, in a patient who had taken an overdose

tissue unless the affected area is treated surgically by skin grafting. An intermediate condition, a 'deep dermal burn' is described where, although some of the dermis still remains viable, it is so small in quantity that spontaneous healing will be slow and imperfect and for the benefit of the patient skin grafting is indicated.

Clinical distinction between superficial and deep burns is important. The superficial burn is a bright mottled red, painful, tender to touch and blanches on pressure from a sterile gauze. It will form blisters and have a profuse fluid loss. The deep burn is a dusky red or even greyish-white, it is insensitive to touch, does not blanch, and is surprisingly painless. There will be much less free flow of fluid from the surface (*Figure 19.1*).

Patients with extensive burns will have some areas of superficial damage, others with full thickness burns and yet others with the intermediate condition of a deep dermal burn.

Biological effects of skin destruction

The skin is the largest single organ in the body. It performs a number of essential biological functions which are lost when the skin is burned. This causes either immediate or long-term complications which vary in severity depending on the extent and the anatomical site of the burn. These vital functions include:

1. *Waterproofing for the body.* As soon as the epidermis is destroyed plasma starts to leak from the burn. If this area is beyond a certain critical percentage of the total body surface, circulatory failure or burns shock will quickly develop unless the lost fluid is replaced by an appropriate infusion.
2. *Baceria-proofing for the body.* Normally pathogenic bacteria in the atmosphere or on the skin do no harm, but if they land on a fresh burn they will rapidly infect it, delay healing and, if untreated, can produce a systemic toxaemia.
3. *Cutaneous sensation.* The skin is a highly developed sensory organ. In a full-thickness burn this function is permanently destroyed. This is particularly serious when the hands are affected.
4. *Elasticity* to allow for distension and movement. Full thickness burns around the rib cage or over joints can have long-term mechanical disadvantages as the scar tissue will contract and limit movement.
5. *Excretory organ.* The skin normally excretes sweat and sebum and if large areas of the skin are replaced by scar tissue or grafts, then the loss of this excretory function becomes important and body temperature regulation may be impaired.

Assessment of a burned patient

It is essential when a burned patient is brought to the Accident and Emergency Department that the doctor who receives the patients knows immediately what to do. The following are the steps to be followed:

1. *Check the airway.* Inhalation of flames, hot gases or smoke can result in oedema developing in the upper respiratory passages and tracheostomy may become necessary. The patient will have sufficient physiological problems without the addition of respiratory

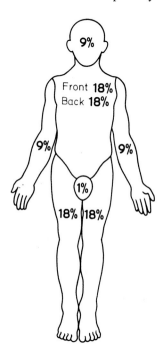

Figure 19.2. Wallace's 'Rule of Nine', for quick assessment of the percentage of the skin which has been injured by burning

obstruction and arrangements should be made early for a planned tracheostomy rather than waiting until the patient is obstructed. Soot in the nostrils or burned nasal hairs are warning signs which must never be neglected.

2. *If the patient is in shock,* establish a reliable intravenous line, take a sample of blood for cross-matching, haematocrit, urea and electrolytes, and start a plasma drip.

3. *If the patient is not in shock,* estimate the percentage of the total skin which is burned. Use Wallace's Rule of Nine (*Figure 19.2*).

Critical limits

In a child or an old person if the percentage burn is 10 per cent or more, or 15 per cent or more in a healthy adult, proceed as in 2 above. If circulatory collapse has not yet occurred it soon will do unless the fluid loss is quickly replaced. These critical limits make intravenous fluid replacement mandatory.

TREATMENT OR PREVENTION OF BURNS SHOCK

This depends on fluid replacement. There are 3 questions to consider:

1. Which fluids to use.
2. How much to give.
3. How quickly to infuse it.

Unfortunately, there is controversy on all these points but a useful and reliable formula for the first few hours is as follows:

total percentage area of the burn × weight in kilograms ÷ 2
= ml of fluid required in each of 6 periods in the first 36 hours
(*Figure 19.3*).

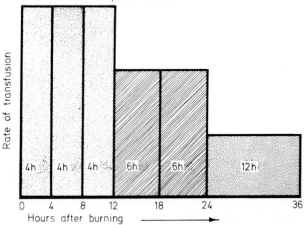

Figure 19.3. The 'Mount Vernon' Transfusion Plan. This gives a forward estimate of the patient's colloid requirement. After the first 4 hours, the actual volume of the transfusion will be modified by the patient's response

Example:

A 60 kg patient with a 30 per cent burn will require $(60 \times 30)/2$ = 900 ml of intravenous fluid in each of the 6 periods, making a total transfusion of 6×900 = 5400 ml within the 36 hours.

It is important to remember that this calculation is to be made from the time of the accident, not from the time when the patient reached hospital. So, if there has been a delay of 2 hours before the patient received treatment, in the above example the patient should receive the first 900 ml within the next 2 hours to put him on schedule.

This formula has proved very satisfactory when the transfusion fluid has been freeze-dried plasma. If Plasma Protein Fraction is used the volume may have to be increased, and if saline or lactated Ringer's solution are used, an even larger increase in the volume is required.

Hourly monitoring of the patient's condition will indicate whether the rate of transfusion requires modification. The following indices are important in this respect:

1. Pulse and blood pressure.
2. Central venous pressure.
3. Jugular vein filling.
4. Pulmonary congestion.
5. Haematocrit.
6. Urine volume and osmolality.

With the widespread catabolic activity which follows an extensive burn a urine output of 0.5–1 ml per minute is necessary to avoid the risk of acute renal failure.

A blood transfusion should form part of the total fluid replacement programme for patients with 10 per cent or more deep burns. A suggested amount is 1 per cent of the patient's normal blood volume for each 1 per cent of deep burn.

Provide analgesia

In full thickness burns where the sensory nerve endings are destroyed this may not be necessary; superficial burns are the more painful. Intravenous morphine 0.2 mg per kilogram body weight diluted in 10 ml of saline and given slowly until the pain is relieved is indicated for large burns. Less extensive burns will cease to be painful when they are hermetically sealed so as to stop evaporation. Neosyn will achieve this for facial burns, Opsite has the same effect for superficial burns on the trunk or extremities.

Management of the burned patient

If the percentage burn is below the critical levels decide whether the patient can be managed as an out-patient or if he still requires in-patient treatment. Factors favouring in-patient treatment are:

1. Suspected respiratory burns.
2. Burns in the perineal region.
3. Full thickness burns which require skin grafting.
4. Poor general health.
5. Poor home circumstances.

In these or other circumstances which require in-patient care the initial treatment of the burn must be given in consultation with the surgeon who will be responsible for the patient while in hospital.

If the percentage burn passes the critical limit, under ideal circumstances, the patient should be transferred to a specialized 'Burns Unit' as soon as the airway is assured, a satisfactory drip started and analgesia given.

Local treatment of the burn

Once the necessary steps have been taken to check the airway, replace fluid and relieve pain, local treatment of the burn consists of a gentle cleaning with cetrimide, removing any remnants of burned clothing and cutting off any strands of dead epithelium which are hanging loose. Small intact blisters may be cleaned and left; large ones, which are likely to burst should be opened with sterile scissors. If the burn is full thickness and passes right round the whole circumference of the trunk, limb or digit, it should be incised longitudinally to prevent occlusion of the circulation or respiratory embarrassment as oedema forms within the burn.

For extensive burns on one aspect only of the trunk or a limb, the 'open-method' of treatment is probably the best. The patient is nursed on a freshly laundered sheet with the burn exposed to light and a current of warm air. In the tropics a mosquito net should be used to keep the flies away. The plasma exuding from the burn will soon coagulate and the coagulum then forms a barrier against further fluid loss and also against infection.

For less extensive superficial burns which can be treated on an out-patient basis, this coagulation can be hastened by using the synthetic produce Neosyn which is made up in a 10 per cent solution of gum acacia. It is applied using a sterile brush and then left to dry. A hair drier will hasten the process and in 20 minutes a child who was brought in screaming, after having pulled a pan of boiling water over its head and neck, will be at ease and may even go off to sleep.

For those parts of the body such as the inner aspects of the arm or legs, where rubbing will break down the coagulum, we have found the application of a sterile sheet of the adhesive plastic film 'Opsite' (Smith & Nephew Pharmaceuticals Ltd) to be very useful (*Figure 19.4*). This application has a further value in that patients can wash over it. As the

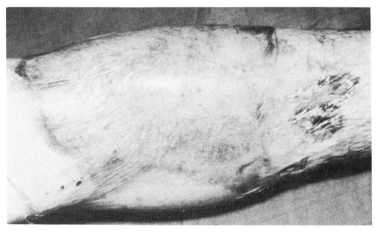

Figure 19.4.   A superficial burn of the leg dressed with 'Opsite'

burn heals beneath it, the Opsite will gradually become detached. For children with burns of the trunk, this method is particularly useful as it avoids using bulky bandages which tend to slip out of place, become soiled and restrict the child's movements.

For small full thickness burns which do not require excision and grafting, and for neglected burns, Flamazine (silver sulphadiazine – Smith & Nephew Pharmaceuticals Ltd) is a useful local application. It is spread liberally over the burn, covered with a tulle dressing and gauze, and secured with bandages.

Once the burn has been effectively dressed it is meddlesome to keep taking the dressing off. The patient should be seen again within 3 to 5 days to ensure that he is comfortable and that the dressing is still satisfactory, and that there are no overt signs of infection. The next visit can then be arranged for a week later, for removal of the dressing. By this time superficial burns should be healed and any necessary further treatment can be considered for deep burns.

Use of antibiotics and tetanus immunization

An extensive study of burns managed on an out-patient basis has shown that only 3 per cent become infected. These few cases can be treated by cetrimide toilet followed by the application of a medicated tulle, for instance Sofratulle (framycetin tulle — Roussel). The use of systemic antibiotics is only indicated in burns extensive enough to require resuscitation.

Patients with deep burns should be immunized against tetanus (*see* Chapter 18).

Prevention of joint contracture

Full thickness or deep dermal burns in the region of joints will, if left to heal naturally, form scar tissue which will then contract and limit the range of movement of the joint. Splinting the joints will diminish this tendency. This is particularly important in the hands which should be supported with the metacarpo-phalangeal joint flexed and the inter-phalangeal joints extended. This position prevents contracture of the collateral ligaments of these joints.

Skin grafting

Patients with full thickness burns, especially if the burn is near a joint, should have the benefit of a plastic surgeon's opinion. Recent trends have been towards applying skin grafts much sooner after the accident. It is preferable for the plastic surgeon to see a patient and decide that grafting will not be necessary than for him to be presented for the first time with a patient with established joint contractures for whom surgery will have to be much more extensive because of delay in seeking surgical replacement of the burned skin (*Figure 19.5*).

BURNS FROM VARIOUS CAUSES

Electricity burns

The burn may be only part of the problem of electrocution. Clearly, if cardiac arrest has occurred, cardio-pulmonary resuscitation takes precedence. The distinctive feature of these burns is that the surface area of

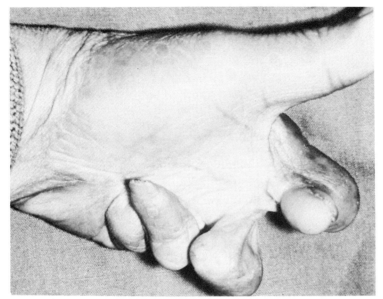

*Figure 19.5. The hand of an Asian immigrant aged 63. She had suffered a burn
injury to her hand when 3 years old*

the burn may be relatively small but there is often a track of dead tissue
along the line of passage of the current. This burn in depth, rather than
in area, creates surgical problems which will often necessitate admission
to hospital and may require surgical treatment for what on the surface,
appears to be a small injury.

Friction burns

These are of two distinct varieties. Firstly, where the patient slides
across an abrading surface, as for instance following a motor cycle
accident, road dirt will be embedded in the burns and must be scrubbed
out under general anaesthesia. Secondly, where some part of the patient
is trapped between moving rollers. Here the skin will be abraded and
scuffed but more important the dermis may have been sheered off the
subcutaneous tissue and so have lost its blood supply. Such a friction
burn may not look too serious when first seen but subsequently there
can be extensive skin necrosis and a plastic surgeon's opinion should be
obtained in the management of these patients.

Chemical burns

The medical and nursing staff working in an A & E Department should be kept informed of any special risks from chemical industries in their locality or of chemical products being regularly transported through their area. Most chemical burns arise in accidents in the home or in school laboratories and can be treated by copious washing with tap water. Corneal burns, after thorough irrigation, should be treated by hydrocortisone drops to diminish the inflammation and possible scarring and be referred for an ophthalmic opinion (*see* Chapter 6).

Radioactivity burns

In Britain comprehensive arrangements for the reception and treatment of patients involved in incidents involving radioactivity are described in the *Health Circular HC(76)52* issued in November 1976, and all Accident Departments should have a copy available for immediate reference.

When the patient is too ill to be taken to one of the specially designated hospitals he will be taken to the nearest A & E Department, and the following advice from the circular should be followed. 'If time is available, the following preparations should be made before the patient arrives at the hospital:

1. An area, not necessarily within the casualty department, should be set aside (the 'dirty' area) for the reception of casualties and, if the floor is not easily cleaned, it should be covered with plastic sheeting or heavy duty paper. Newspaper can be used if nothing else is available.
2. Protective clothing should be issued for all staff who will handle the patient.
3. A plentiful supply of paper towels and tissue should be available.
4. Large polythene or paper bags will be needed for the collection of the patient's clothing and contaminated equipment etc.
5. An area should be cleared where the ambulance can wait for monitoring and possible decontamination.
6. A limited number of staff should be appointed to handle the patient and a person should be designated to log the movements of any of those staff who must leave the 'dirty' area after the casualties have arrived, in order to minimize the difficulty of tracing contamination.
7. If other areas of the hospital become involved in handling the patient, e.g. a theatre or Intensive Care Unit, similar arrangements should be made for these areas as appropriate.

8. A person should be designated to deal with enquiries, public relations, etc.

The following initial decontamination procedures should be followed:

1. Experience has shown that washing with soap and water will effectively remove contaminated material from the skin in most cases. Initial treatment and any necessary washing to remove as much of the suspected contamination as practicable should be done in the 'dirty' area.
2. Open wounds should be irrigated. Special care needs to be taken in the cleaning of areas near the eyes and in preventing the spread of possible contamination to other parts of the body.
3. It will usually be possible to seek further expert advice from a designated hospital before proceeding beyond the initial treatment stage, and it is inadvisable to excise wounds, unless contamination is obvious or unless surgically indicated, before monitoring assistance is available.'

20

The Treatment of the Acute Abscess

BASIC PATHOLOGY OF ABSCESS FORMATION AND RESPONSE TO TREATMENT

An abscess if a collection of pus surrounded by a pyogenic membrane. As the abscess grows in size the inner surface of the membrane sloughs and liquifies to add to the volume of pus, and the outer surface enlarges as the body continues the battle to localize and contain the area of infection. The membrane has two important properties: it prevents the spread of toxic products or live bacteria from the abscess into the general circulation and it allows leucocytes to pass from the circulation into the abscess to ingest the bacteria. Unfortunately, from the point of view of therapy, antibiotics carried in the blood stream do not traverse the pyogenic membrane and so cannot play any direct role in the treatment of an abscess unless this barrier is first breached by surgical intervention.

Before the advent of antibiotics it was common surgical practice to delay incision of an abscess until it was bulging under the skin. To hasten this process, poltices or formentations were used to 'draw' the abscess to the surface. Then, once it was 'ripe' or 'pointing', it was realized from empirical observation that incision would allow the pus to drain away without infecting the surrounding tissues. At the beginning of the antibiotic era Maurice Ellis showed that if an intramuscular injection of an effective antibiotic was given ½ to 1 hour before incision, the risk of spreading the infection to surrounding tissues, by operating early in the evolution of the abscess, was completely eradicated. Consequently, poltices and formentations were no longer needed and they now have no role to play in the modern treatment of an acute abscess. If pus is judged to be present, arrangements should be made immediately to let it out under an antibiotic cover.

Ellis continued this pioneer work by showing that if, at the time of incision of an acute abscess, the pus was thoroughly evacuated, any loculi were broken down and all slough and dead tissue removed, then, using a curette, the pyogenic membrane was scraped out, and antibiotic-laden blood would fill the cavity. This resulted in the area being rendered aseptic and so permitted the surgeon to perform a primary closure. Prior to this advance in surgical technique a surgeon, having evacuated the pus from an abscess cavity, felt obliged to pack the cavity with a 'wick' or ribbon gauze to prevent the cavity closing at the surface before the deeper portion had healed. The essential point in the Ellis technique is that the cavity should be occluded by deep sutures passing right round it to obliterate any dead space. Healing then takes place simultaneously throughout the whole area of the former abscess.

A further advantage of this technique is that, as all the cellular and humeral elements necessary for wound healing are already on site in abundance, there is no lag phase in the speed of wound healing. Whereas a clean surgical incision may require 8 days before the sutures can be safely removed, an incision in a formerly infected, but now sterile area, will heal in 5 days. Provided the surgery is correctly performed and the antibiotic is effective against the causal organism, the treatment can be used on an out-patient basis. Under optimum conditions the patient only makes 2 visits to hospital, one for the initial surgery, and the second to have the sutures removed after 5 days. Healing will be delayed in those patients who waited until the abscess was 'pointing' before coming for treatment. The same technique is applicable but there will be some superficial skin necrosis, the skin having been damaged by the inflammatory process. If pointing has proceeded to actual bursting through the skin, a small abscess will then heal spontaneously but a large one still justifies a full surgical curettage and suture under anti-biotic cover, otherwise a sinus may result from the small opening usually present. Failure of this technique to produce rapid and complete healing usually means that one or more of the following errors has been committed:

1. The antibiotic has inadvertently been forgotten.
2. All loculi were not broken down.
3. Slough, dead tissue or pyogenic membrane were left in the cavity.
4. The sutures did not adequately obliterate the cavity.
5. The organisms were insensitive to the antibiotic.

SPECIAL SITES OF ABSCESS FORMATION

Infection in the hand

Delay in operating on abscesses in the infected hand is still far too common. Very early infection of the hand before a definite abscess is formed may respond to antibiotic treatment. However, if the patient's sleep has been disturbed the previous night by a throbbing pain in the hand, pus is almost certainly present and incision under an antibiotic cover should be planned immediately. Physical examination will show the classical signs of local heat, redness, pain and swelling, and occasionally the added complications of lymphangitis and axillary lymphadenitis. If the patient gives a history of frequent soft tissue infection, his general health should be investigated. Diabetes, leukaemia or an underlying focus of infection such as osteomyelitis must be considered. Asian immigrants in Britain frequently present with a rapidly evolving tuberculous infection of the soft tissues which fortunately responds quickly to appropriate antibiotic treatment once the correct diagnosis is made.

Anaesthesia

For infections in the distal half of a finger a digital nerve block is indicated: 2 ml of 1 per cent lignocaine, without adrenaline, are injected into the region of the digital nerves at the base of the finger. These nerves run on each side of the finger mid-way between palmar and dorsal aspects. After injection it may take up to 15 minutes for the anaesthetic to penetrate to the centre of the nerve and so anaesthetize the sensory fibres which arise at the finger tip. For more proximally situated infections in the hand, general or regional anaesthesia is necessary.

Paronychia

This very common condition, an infection at the side of the nail, commonly called a 'whitlow' may arise from three separate causes: usually bacterial, occasionally fungal and very occasionally viral.

Acute paronychia.   This is usually due to a staphylococcal infection. To effect a cure under a digital block, an incision is made parallel to the edge of the nail and 1 mm away from it. A swab is taken from the pus, pyogenic membrane and any dead tissue are curetted away and then the wound edges will fall into place. A firm dressing will obliterate any dead space. The condition is usually fully healed in 4 days.

Sub-acute paronychia.   This condition has usually been present for 2 to 3 weeks before the patient seeks treatment and it is not as painful as acute paronychia. The cause is a fungus infection which will respond to applications of an anti-fungal ointment and an occlusive dressing.

'Herpetic whitlow'

This is an occupational hazard of nurses, especially those nursing tracheostomy patients. Nurses doing tracheal toilet or dressings should wear disposable gloves. The lesion starts as a vesicle surrounded by inflammation. In succeeding days further vesicles appear and the condition becomes increasingly painful. Incision will fail to demon-

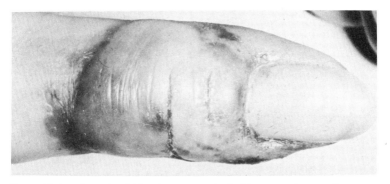

Figure 20.1.   Herpetic whitlow in a nurse who had been treating a tracheostomy patient. Surgical treatment does not help this condition

strate any pus but may result in secondary bacterial infection. Antibiotics have no effect on the virus and the only treatment is to dress the finger with idoxuridine which will ease the pain and speed up healing (*Figure 20.1*).

Pulp space infections

These are extremely painful. The soft tissues and skin which form the pulp at the ends of the fingers have a very rich sensory innervation; consequently, patients tend to come early for treatment. A surgical approach should be made from the dorsal aspect under cover of the hood of the projecting finger nail. In this way scarring across the sensitive skin of the pulp is avoided. All dead tissue must be carefully removed because any lingering infection may result in infection spreading to the bone of the terminal phalanx and producing an osteomyelitis. After adequate surgery, suturing is rarely necessary; a firm dressing will hold the tissues in place and occlude any dead space. Healing should be complete within a week.

Subcutaneous abscess

These abscesses can occur anywhere on the fingers or hand and the acute paronychia and pulp space infections are no more than a subcutaneous abscess in a particularly common site. The principles of treatment are the same. Incision should be made in the line of the skin creases and care must be taken to evacuate all the pus. Occasionally a 'collar stud' abscess may develop with superficial and deep pockets of pus connected only by a narrow sinus. If only the superficial pus is evacuated the condition will fail to respond to the treatment.

Web space infection

This infection occurs at the base of the finger on the palmar aspect. The infection spreads quickly into the webs of the finger, proximally into the palm for about 2 cm, and distally into the proximal segment of the finger. Redness and oedema usually develop early on the dorsum of the hand. Indeed, the patient often shows the red swollen dorsum of the hand as the main area of complaint, but questioning and physical examination will establish that the centre of infection is on the palmar aspect at the base of the finger. Under general anaesthesia an incision is made in the proximal palmar crease of the finger, care being taken not to incise too deeply and involve the flexor tendon sheath (*Figure 20.2*). After squeezing out the pus and curetting the lining of the abscess, a firm dressing is applied because the natural semi-flexed position of the fingers apposes the skin edges and collapses the cavity. Healing will be complete in 4 to 5 days, whereas if an incision is made in the finger web, even if it is sutured, it would take well over a week to heal.

Suppurative tenosynovitis

This condition is now rare in Britain but when it occurs the treatment is important and urgent. In the early stages pus develops in the fibrous flexor sheath of a finger. Gradually the tension in the sheath equals or exceeds the pressure in the surrounding arterioles and capillaries and the blood supply to the tendons is occluded. If the sheath is not promptly decompressed, the tendons undergo necrosis and the patient is left with a useless stiff finger. The usual presentation is of a painful, throbbing, tender, sausage-shaped swelling on the volar aspect of the finger extending into the distal half of the palm. The finger is held semi-flexed, extension of the finger is painful and further flexion is limited by the swelling. Treatment should be given under general anaesthesia

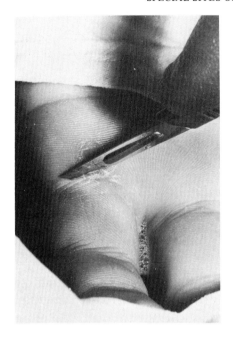

Figure 20.2. A superficial incision in the line of the proximal flexor crease of a finger is used to decompress and curette a web space infection

and a tourniquet. After a pre-operative intramuscular injection of an effective antibiotic, one incision is made in the mid-palmar crease and a second one in the flexor crease of the distal interphalangeal joint. This allows the flexor sheath to be opened both proximally and distally. A No. 4 FG plastic catheter is now passed along the sheath to decompress it and to irrigate it with an antibiotic solution. Once a free flow of the antibiotic solution has been established the catheter can be withdrawn and the incisions closed. Antibiotic therapy should be continued orally for 4 to 5 days by which time the symptoms should have resolved, but the patient may benefit from wax baths and exercises in the Physiotherapy Department to help him regain full use of the finger.

Palmar space infections

Infections localized to the thenar, mid-palmar or hypothenar spaces are now very rarely seen. They probably only arise as a complication of a neglected or inadequately treated infection elsewhere in the hand. The principles of treatment are the same: incision and curettage under an antibiotic cover followed by oral antibiotic therapy.

Carbuncle

This type of infection occurs on the dorsum of the hand and fingers in association with hair follicles. Antibiotics will not heal the condition but may prevent the infection spreading to other adjacent hair follicles. A hygroscopic dressing such as magnesium sulphate paste will help to draw the pus and slough out of the follicles. If resolution is slow surgical removal of the slough is indicated.

Abscesses of the neck

There are two common varieties of abscess in the neck: a suppurative lymphadenitis in a deep cervical lymph gland and an alveolar abscess arising from the inner surface of the mandible. It is often difficult when palpating these swellings to be certain that pus is present. Examination is made difficult because the patient is usually a young child who objects vigorously to anyone touching the swelling. Experience has shown that when the skin over the swelling is at all red, pus is present. On incision the alveolar abscess is usually surrounded by a mass of indurated tissue and careful blunt dissection is required to release the few millimetres of pus at the centre of the inflammatory mass. Once the pus has been cleared away with a curette or gauze, no pack or drain is required. Even though the anatomical site precludes the use of an obliterating deep suture, provided effective antibiotic therapy is given, the wound will have healed and the inflammation resolved in 4 to 5 days.

Axillary abscesses

These are very common especially in patients who shave the axilla and use a deodorant. The Ellis treatment of incision, curettage and primary sutures under an antibiotic cover is eminently suitable and, provided it is properly executed, there is no place for the use of packs or wicks which, being in themselves foreign bodies, can only serve to delay healing.

Breast abscesses

The incidence of this abscess has declined greatly in the last decade, probably because of improved methods of suppressing lactation in the post-partum period. Because of the amenable anatomical structure of the breast, the Ellis treatment probably benefits these patients more than any others. A large breast abscess may contain 50–100 ml of pus and an enthusiastic but ill-informed surgeon can pack the cavity with several metres of ribbon gauze. When, in 3 or 4 days' time, the patient is submitted to the painful experience of changing the pack, the surgeon may be pleased to see some slight further drainage of pus and will remark 'the abscess is draining freely now'. It is our contention that he should say to himself 'due to the foreign vegetable matter I have introduced into this patient in the form of a cotton wick, I have stimulated the production of laudable pus much as did my illustrious predecessors in the eighteenth century when they buried peas or beans in the wound'. Packing a breast abscess in this way can perpetuate it for weeks. Using the Ellis technique, with an incision radiating away from the nipple followed by a comprehensive curettage, the abscess will heal in 5 days, especially because the breast is so amenable to the use of deep obliterative sutures. There can be no doubt that this method should be used in all acute breast abscesses.

Occasionally a rapidly growing, anaplastic carcinoma of breast may look line an abscess. If, on incision, no pus is found but rather tumour-like tissue and necrotic fluid, a biopsy should be taken and further surgical advice obtained.

Ano-rectal abscesses

This common condition has provided the most testing challenge to the Ellis technique of abscess treatment and it is this type of abscess which has been most thoroughly investigated in assessing the value of the method. The patient is usually middle-aged (30–50) and comes to the Accident and Emergency Department complaining of a throbbing, painful swelling around the anus which has kept him awake for the past 2 or 3 nights. The physical signs depend on the degree of evolution of the abscess. In the early stages, there may be nothing more than an area of tender induration but, if sleep has been disturbed, pus is present and surgery should be arranged immediately.

The traditional method of treatment for this abscess is to make an incision radiating away from the anal orifice to release the pus, then to de-roof the cavity by making a second incision at right-angles to the first one. The edges of the skin are trimmed with scissors and haemostasis achieved using diathermy coagulation; the cavity is then packed with ribbon gauze soaked in an antiseptic solution. Post-operatively the patient remains in hospital and the pack is changed daily until healing is sufficiently advanced in 5 or 6 days' time for subsequent dressings to be done by the District Nurse or by the patient himself at home.

Using the Ellis method, the patients are treated on an out-patient basis but the surgical procedure requires at least as much care and operative skill as does the traditional method. Half to one hour before surgery, the patient is given an intramuscular injection of an antibiotic. The choice of antibiotic is important: it must be effective against anaerobic organisms such as bacteriodes as well as the staphylococcus because a variety of organisms can be responsible for the infection. Then, under a general anaesthetic the patient is placed in the lithotomy position, the perineum is shaved and a sigmoidoscope passed to detect any communication between the abscess and the lumen of the bowel. If such a communication is found the condition is then, by definition, a fistula-in-ano and primary closure will no longer be applicable. Assuming that this unusual complication is not present, a radial incision is made, a bacteriological swab is taken of the first pus to flow out, and the gloved index finger inserted to determine whether the abscess is 'perianal' with an intact ischio-rectal fascia above it, or 'ischio-rectal' with a perforation of the fascia. In the latter instance, this perforation must be enlarged to allow complete evacuation of the pus and pyogenic membrane lying above the fascia. After thorough curettage all remaining debris is removed by a gauze toilet of the cavity. Then, using a 2/0 monofilament nylon suture on a large half circle needle, the left index finger is placed in the cavity to gauge the depth to which the sutures must be passed to occlude the cavity; 2 or 3 sutures are introduced before any are tied. Finally, a sterile dressing is applied and after recovering from the anaesthetic the patient can return home with a 4-day course of oral antibiotic. If the dressing becomes soiled it can be changed at home or at the hospital. On the fifth or sixth day the wound is inspected. Usually by this time, because all the swelling has subsided, the sutures are lying loose and can be easily removed. The patient may now be discharged or may require one further out-patient visit for a final removal of the dressing.

We have previously published a retrospective 2-year follow-up of 100 patients treated in this way. This showed a 78 per cent success rate without any recurrence of symptoms, 15 per cent of patients had another abscess form within the succeeding 2 years, and 7 per cent developed

Table 20.1

COMPARISON OF THE RESULTS OF A RANDOMIZED TRIAL OF THE
TREATMENT OF ANO-RECTAL ABSCESS (see TEXT)

	Traditional method	Ellis method
Number of patients	109	110
Average no. of days as an in-patient	4	0
Average no. of days off work	31	8
Average no. of days to full healing	35	10

an anal fistula. More recently we have co-operated with Leaper *et al*. in a prospective study of 219 patients treated on a randomized basis either by the traditional method or by the Ellis method. *Table 20.1* indicates the advantages for the patient of the Ellis method.

References

Ellis, M. (1960). Incision and primary suture of abscesses of the anal region, *Proc. R. Soc. Med.,* 53, 652

Leaper, D. J., Page, R. E., Rosenberg, I. L., Wilson, D. H. & Goliger, J. C. (1976). A controlled study comparing the conventional treatment of idiopathic ano-rectal abscess with that of incision, curettage and primary suture under systemic antibiotic cover, *Dis. Colon Rectum*, 19 (1), 46

Wilson, D. H. (1964). The late results of ano-rectal abscess treated by incision, curettage and primary suture under antibiotic cover, *Br. J. Surg.*, 51, 828

21

The Acute Abdomen

The diagnosis of acute surgical disease in the abdomen forms one of the most fascinating parts of the work of the Emergency Department. Abdominal pain may be accompanied by other symptoms such as fever, nausea or vomiting, diarrhoea or frequency of micturition, but it is usually the pain which is the presenting symptom. A careful history and examination, and certain basic investigations are required to diagnose or exclude an acute surgical cause for the pain. With years of experience a senior doctor will improve his diagnostic acumen, learning which questions to ask and how much significance to attach to the answers. A junior doctor, especially if working under pressure or through the night hours, is more likely to make a wrong decision which could have disastrous consequences for the patient.

A recent study of the diagnostic accuracy of junior doctors working unaided in an Accident and Emergency Department showed that their provisional diagnosis was correct for only 42 per cent of patients admitted to hospital with an 'acute abdomen' (Wilson, D. H., Wilson, P. D., Walmsley, R. G., Horrocks, J. C. and de Dombal, F. T., 1977, *Br. J. Surg.*, **64**, 250). The introduction of an 'Acute Abdominal Chart' or diagnostic check-list (*Figure 21.1*) enabled them to develop a systematized method of history-taking and physical examination of a patient with acute abdominal symptoms, and to avoid forgetting to ask certain essential questions. Once the final diagnosis is established, the completed chart is returned to the Emergency Department to provide 'feed-back' information and to permit further discussion and tuition in areas of diagnostic weakness. The immediate results of this innovation were to raise the diagnostic accuracy of the doctors who made the initial examination from 42 per cent to 61 per cent and also to increase significantly their ability to send a patient home with a confident and correct decision that their symptoms did not require hospital treatment.

In Leeds it has been shown that it is practical to use a computer to store the diagnostic information gained from many hundreds of patients with acute abdominal disease. Then the details of the signs and symptoms

ACUTE ABDOMINAL CHART

NAME:		CASUALTY NUMBER:
AGE:	SEX:	CASUALTY OFFICER:
PRESENTATION (999, GP, etc.):		DATE/TIME:

HISTORY	EXAMINATION

PRESENTING SYMPTOM(S)

GENERAL
Mood:
Colour:

Temp:
Pulse:
Resp:
B.P.:

PAIN
Site at onset   Site at present
Severity
Aggravating factors
Relieving factors
Progress
Duration
Type of pain

ABDOMINAL
Movement
Scars
Distension

Tenderness (indicate)

Rebound
Guarding
Rigidity
Murphy's sign
Swellings
Bowel sounds
Rectal examination
Vaginal examination

OTHER SYMPTOMS
Nausea
Vomiting
Anorexia
Weight
Previous indigestion
Jaundice
Bowels
Micturition
Female { Periods
          { Vag. discharge
          { Pregnancy

INITIAL DIAGNOSIS AND PLAN:

PAST MEDICAL HISTORY
Previous similar pain

Previous operations

Previous illnesses

Drugs
Allergies

OTHER CLINICAL DATA

INVESTIGATIONS
Blood count:
Urine:
X-Ray:
Other:

DIAGNOSIS AFTER INVESTIGATION: FINAL DIAGNOSIS:

TREATMENT: OUTCOME:

Figure 21.1.   Diagnostic check-list currently in use in the General Infirmay at Leeds. It is designed for computer analysis of the diagnostic information. This version of the form is being used to assess the value of investigation in the Emergency Department

from new patients can be compared with this data base and the computer will make a diagnostic prediction which is at least as reliable as that of the most experienced clinician. We are not suggesting that the computer can replace the clinician, but we do consider that it can be of great help in improving the level of diagnostic accuracy.

In ideal circumstances, quite apart from these methods, a junior doctor should be present in the theatre when a patient's abdomen is explored so that he can see for himself the significance of the signs and symptoms he has elicited.

ACUTE APPENDICITIS

In temperate climes, the commonest acute surgical lesion producing abdominal pain is acute appendicitis. The population at large, particularly anxious mothers and school teachers, nearly always think of appendicitis as the cause of abdominal pain, especially if the pain is on the right side. In the study referred to on page 204, of 1196 consecutive patients presenting at the General Infirmary at Leeds with undiagnosed abdominal pain of less than 1 week's duration, only 187 (or 15.6 per cent) were found to have acute appendicitis. The total of all other patients requiring urgent surgery was just under 10 per cent so, although acute appendicitis patients are only 1 in 6 or 7 of all patients with acute abdominal pain, nevertheless they clearly exceed the total of all other patients requiring immediate operation. Sifting out those patients who require urgent surgical treatment from those who merit observation in hospital and from those who can be safely sent home, is a continuing challenge.

Clinical picture

The standard, classical picture of acute appendicitis is that of:

1. Central abdominal pain; followed by:
2. Nausea or vomiting; followed by:
3. Localization of the pain in the right iliac fossa with localized tenderness.

Many cases do not fit into this neat picture, and all factors shown on the abdominal chart must be considered in turn.

Age

Acute appendicitis is predominantly a young person's disease and when it occurs in a small child or an old person, it is more difficult to diagnose. Intussusception in the child and malignancy in the elderly are possible alternative diagnoses. In geriatric patients the condition may proceed to peritonitis and even then they may still have a soft abdomen.

Sex

In young female patients 'Mittelschmerz', or the pain of ovulation in the middle of the menstrual cycle may, for a few hours, mimic appendicitis. The pain of salpingitis is felt in the pelvic region from the beginning and vaginal examination will confirm the presence of a tender swollen fallopian tube. Similarly, a right-sided tubal abortion should be distinguishable from appendicitis especially if there is the added history of a missed period. A twisted right ovarian cyst is usually much more painful than an early appendicitis and the absence of a raised temperature will also favour this diagnosis even though the cyst may not be easy to feel. Acute appendicitis occurring in the last trimestre of pregnancy may be confusing and difficult to manage and the advice of an experienced obstetrician will be helpful.

Presenting symptom

Pain should always be the first and the dominant symptom in acute appendicitis. Vomiting or diarrhoea as the first symptom make the diagnosis of acute appendicitis unlikely, and headache as the first symptom virtually excludes it.

Duration of pain

Diagnosis of acute appendicitis within 3 hours of onset of pain has been made correctly, but 6–8 hours is usually required for certainty. At the other extreme, after 48 hours one of 3 things is happening if the disease is acute appendicitis:

1. The patient is getting better.
2. Peritonitis is developing.
3. An appendix abscess is forming.

If none of these events has happened, appendicitis becomes the least probable cause of the abdominal pain. Physical examination should confirm or exclude peritonitis or a lump in the right iliac fossa and, as the patient has come to hospital, it is unlikely that he is getting better.

Type of pain

In appendicitis the pain may be colicky or a throbbing inflammatory pain. The severity of the pain may wax and wane. If the pain is truly intermittent, with periods of complete freedom between attacks, appendicitis is most unlikely, with one exception. In many cases of appendix abscess, quite a large lump may be present with the patient giving a clear history of a period of complete freedom from pain, eating normally and following his usual activities. If, however, after careful examination no lump is discovered, intermittent pain should mean no appendicitis.

Other symptoms

Nausea, vomiting, anorexia, diarrhoea or constipation, frequency of micturition and dysuria may occur and their presence should be noted. Their presence or absence is only 'fringe' evidence in the diagnosis of appendicitis and the assessment of their significance should await the results of the physical examination. Vomiting before onset of pain is against the diagnosis of appendicitis. Too much should not be made of this in children, for the onset of pain and vomiting are often so close together that it is hard for the child to say which came first.

Physical examination

Temperature, pulse and respiration

These should be recorded as routine. Commonly in appendicitis, the temperature is between 37.5 and 38.0°C and the pulse rate between 80 and 90 per minute. Absence of pyrexia or a pulse rated between 70 and 80 do not rule out appendicitis.

At the other extreme, a temperature well above 38°C is of significance. Uncomplicated acute appendicitis does not produce high pyrexia. A temperature of 39°C or more means either that the appendicitis has become complicated by peritonitis or an abscess, or that the cause of the symptoms is something other than appendicitis. A useful rule is that if the temperature exceeds 38°C, in the absence of peritonitis or an abscess, a search should be made for some other cause of the pain.

Mood

In uncomplicated appendicitis the patient is not usually very distressed. A flush on the cheeks, chin and brow means either that peritonitis is present, or that the pain is not caused by appendicitis. The grey face of patients with advanced peritonitis once seen is always remembered; they look and feel as though death is near.

Abdominal examination

The history together with the preliminary examination, have so far only suggested the possibilities of diagnosis. The final diagnosis awaits the findings on physical examination of the abdomen. This examination should be gentle and unhurried. It is best to sit by the examination couch or bedside. The hands must be warm, if necessary wash them in warm water. The patient must be lying flat, with a suitable pillow under the head, and with hips and knees slightly flexed. The abdomen must be completely exposed for examination.

Inspection.   The presence of abdominal scars will prompt a question about previous illness and operation, if this has not been done already. Remember that post-operative adhesions are the commonest cause of intestinal obstruction and if the appendix was removed at a previous laparotomy it cannot now be the cause of pain. Uncomplicated appendicitis does not produce a distended abdomen. Blowing the abdomen out and pulling it in flat can be done, but are painful in appendicitis. An obvious lump in the right iliac fossa in a thin abdomen may be an appendix abscess.

Palpation.   This is carried out gently to discover tenderness, rigidity or a lump. The pressure on the abdominal wall should at first be light and then gradually increased so that the depths of the abdomen are felt. Begin in the left iliac fossa and work cautiously round to reach the right iliac fossa last. Since tenderness is due to direct pressure on the inflamed appendix, deep palpation will be necessary when the appendix is retrocaecal. Because the appendix has length and breadth, the area of tenderness in acute appendicitis has length and breadth. This area is usually covered by the tips of 3 fingers. In acute appendicitis palpation to one side or other, above or below this area, produces minimal or no tenderness. A return to the 'guilty' area will again produce tenderness. The discovery of this tenderness, constant in position and severity, clinches the diagnosis of acute appendicitis.

If peritonitis is present, severe tenderness will be found to be more widespread and there will be rigidity of the overlying muscles producing local guarding. If there is a lump, careful palpation should reveal its presence and size.

Palpation of the abdomen may, however, reveal no localized tenderness, no widespread tenderness, no rigidity and no lump. All that is discovered is a vague tenderness, possibly at its maximum on the right lower abdomen. A rectal examination should now be made. The object is to discover a tender mass in the rectovesical pouch or pouch of Douglas in the female. The discovery of this tender mass, together with the history already elicited, makes the diagnosis of pelvic abscess probably due to appendicitis.

When rectal examination produces nothing abnormal, we are left with the abdominal findings of vague, generalized tenderness. We can now say that if:

1. the time elapsed since the onset of symptoms exceeds 48 hours;
or
2. the temperature exceeds 38°C;

then the cause of the pain is probably not acute appendicitis.

Differential diagnoses

While remembering that common things occur commonly and that a case of acute appendicitis should never be missed, there are other diagnoses which may be confused with appendicitis. Lower lobe pneumonia or pleurisy on the right side of the chest may simulate the pain of appendicitis, but physical examination and a chest X-ray should clearly distinguish between the two. Myocardial infarction is an increasingly common cause of acute pain and its occurrence is increasing in young middle-aged people. Even though the description of the pain may be vague and the radiation bizarre a careful history and physical examination should avoid any confusion with appendicitis. Perforated peptic ulcer, acute cholecystitis and intestinal obstruction are discussed later in this chapter.

The diarrhoea and vomiting or gastro-enteritis may produce severe spasms of abdominal pain with an intermittent dull ache and generalized tenderness over the abdomen. In children a pelvic appendicitis may produce diarrhoea, but the rectal examination should establish this diagnosis. An inflamed appendix lying close to the urinary tract may, by inflammatory irritation, produce frequency and dysuria. Tenderness in the loin or a tender palpable kidney with heavily infected urine will suggest pyelitis rather than appendicitis as the cause of these urinary symptoms.

Negro children with sickle cell disease may suffer from acute abdominal pain due to small mesenteric infarcts, and older people with arteriosclerosis may have larger infarcts producing intestinal obstruction. Drug addicts may simulate the pain of acute appendicitis or other abdominal disease. Their insistent demands for an analgesic injection should raise one's suspicion. If there is a previous operation scar a gesture at ringing the previous hospital for further information often precipitates their prompt departure.

The main diagnostic problem is to distinguish between appendicitis and the non-specific abdominal pain which some authors attribute to mesenteric lymphadenitis. These latter patients are usually children aged 12 years or less, their pain is intermittent and they are free of pain between attacks. They may recently have had an upper respiratory tract infection and there may be enlarged, tender cervical lymph nodes. If after examination the diagnosis is still in doubt, 3 or 4 hours in the observation ward will suffice to clear up the doubt. In the appendicitis patient the symptoms progress, while the symptoms of the patient with non-specific abdominal pain remain stationary or recede and they can be safely returned home, with strict instructions to return to hospital if the symptoms recur — it is very rare for them to do so.

INTESTINAL OBSTRUCTION

The majority of patients with intestinal obstruction present themselves to the doctor because of pain. There is a smaller group of patients for whom vomiting is the principal complaint.

Clinical features

The pain is colicky, coming on intermittently. In adults this pain is rarely of comparable severity with that of renal colic. A history of intermittent abdominal pain should raise the suspicion of intestinal obstruction and other symptoms must be sought to confirm or refute this diagnosis.

Vomiting

If vomiting is present as well as recurring colicky pain, it is certainly confirmatory evidence, but the absence of vomiting or only trivial vomiting does not rule out obstruction. Vomiting may be quite late in appearance with obstruction at the lower end of the large bowel, but can be a very early symptom in proximal small bowel obstruction.

Constipation

If present, this again is confirmatory evidence, but its absence does not rule out obstruction especially when the site of the lesion is in the small bowel. It is always necessary to enquire about it or a patient with colicky pain and vomiting may omit to mention that he has diarrhoea and thus a case of gastro-enteritis may be mis-diagnosed as obstruction, especially as in the severe case fluid levels may be seen on X-ray.

In obstruction then, we may have recurring colicky pain with vomiting but no constipation, or the pain with constipation but little or no vomiting. In either case we should be able to diagnose the obstruction before the late, third symptom develops. The patient may volunteer that there is a painful swelling, suggesting a strangulated hernia as the cause of the obstruction, but the absence of a painful lump does not rule out the diagnosis of obstruction. Intestinal adhesions, mesenteric infarction, volvulus, an internal hernia, tumour or, in the elderly diverticulitis or chronic constipation may be the cause.

Physical examination

The suspicion of intestinal obstruction having been raised by the history, the abdomen is examined with the patient lying flat with a pillow under the head, and the hips and knees slightly flexed. The whole of the abdomen must be uncovered or the presence of a lump around the groins may be missed. A small femoral hernia in a corpulent female is easily overlooked. A quick inspection of the groins may show an obvious lump, but at this stage palpation should wait. Inspection is an important part of the examination. With obstruction, the abdomen is always distended to a greater or lesser degree and, excluding a strangulated hernia with a painful, tender external lump, obstruction cannot really be diagnosed without distension. But the distension of obstruction is caused by gas in coils of gut, and since all coils are not equally distended with gas, the distension of the abdomen will be asymmetrical. With a history of intermittent colicky pain with vomiting or constipation, as soon as the abdomen is uncovered look for irregular distension. If it is present, sit down and watch it. After a while the irregular pattern will alter: small mounds of distension will appear which were not there a minute before, while other distended mounds will disappear. The period of observation need not be longer than 5 minutes at the outside to be sure that these changes in distension are taking place. Further physical examination is aimed at finding out the cause of the obstruction. After palpation of the groins, loins and abdomen, rectal examination is a mandatory part of the examination. In old people this can reveal a mass of impacted faeces, which may be the size of a cricket ball. In these cases, manual evacuation, if necessary under anaesthetic, is followed by a dramatic recovery. In other patients rectal examination may reveal a tumour as the cause of the obstruction, or the rectum may be dilated and empty, which is confirmatory evidence of the diagnosis already made.

Radiological examination

This should follow the completion of the physical examination and is never a substitute for it. Two views are taken: one with the patient supine and one in the erect position. The appearance of fluid levels on the erect film, except for a patient with severe gastro-enteritis or a child under 2 years of age, are confirmatory evidence of intestinal obstruction. Volvulae conniventes seen to traverse the full diameter of the small bowel or the appearance of haustrations on the large bowel are further confirmatory radiological signs.

All patients with intestinal obstruction require urgent admission to hospital and they usually require a laparotomy.

INTUSSUSCEPTION

These cases are often very difficult to diagnose. The typical case occurs in an infant around the age of 1 year. Boys are affected more often than girls. The baby cannot complain of pain, but the mother seeks help because, from out of the blue, the infant has an attack of screaming as if it were in pain. There may be vomiting and there may be the passage of the classical redcurrant jelly motions. Vomiting is so frequent with any sick infant that no special diagnostic weight can be attached to it. The 'redcurrant jelly' passed per rectum makes the diagnosis of intussusception very probable, but some forms of gastro-enteritis can produce this, as can bacillary dissentery, which is common in tropical countries.

Usually with intussusception, the child looks quite well between the attacks of screaming. By contrast, the child with gastro-enteritis or dysentry looks toxic, especially if the symptoms have persisted for 24 hours or more. Attempting to examine the abdomen of a restless crying child will probably not reveal any valuable information. The examiner must use all his wits to see that the child is lying relaxed and quiet. It usually pays to tell the mother exactly what is required. Playing with the child, nursing it or talking to it may not succeed. The doctor should leave the room and come back quietly when the child is relaxed and then place a warm gentle hand on the abdomen to feel for the typical sausage-shaped lump. The lump is usually palpable in the epigastrium and may be felt as soon as the hand is placed there. If it is not felt immediately, the hand should stay there and wait. After a short time, if there is an intussusception, a wave of peristalsis will make the gut contract and the tumour will be felt. Only too often just as the peristalsis comes on the child feels pain, starts to cry, the abdominal wall contracts and the chance of feeling the tumour goes. The examination may have to be repeated several times, but if there is an intussusception, a tumour can usually be felt eventually and the diagnosis established.

Only when the abdominal examination is complete should a rectal examination be performed. If there has already been a redcurrant jelly motion, it is not really necessary. Sometimes some of this characteristic stool is seen on the tip of the examining finger. Occasionally the apex of the intussusception may be palpated in the rectum.

A skilled radiologist will be able to help when the diagnosis is in doubt by giving a barium enema and occasionally, in an early case, the enema can be used as a means of therapy to reduce the intussusception.

PERFORATED PEPTIC ULCER

The diagnosis of the typical perforated peptic ulcer is one of the easiest to make of all the acute abdominal catastropes. A history of severe abdominal pain of recent onset, combined with generalized abdominal tenderness and board-like rigidity of the abdominal muscles, makes an unmistakable clinical picture. The patient lies immobile and the typical steely grey facies, once recognized, suggests the diagnosis as the doctor approaches the bedside. As these perforations can occur at any time, the severity of the pain may cause the patient to come to hospital from home, the street or from work without waiting to be seen by the general practitioner.

The more difficult case is the patient who is known to have a duodenal ulcer of longstanding and who comes to hospital with a severe exacerbation of pain often after imbibing a quantity of alcohol. In some of these patients, the ulcer has perforated and the typical picture described above is present. In others there has only been a small localized leak of duodenal contents which is then sealed off by the omentum and surrounding viscera. Radiological examination may be particularly help-ful in determining the diagnosis for these patients. The film of the abdomen taken in the erect position will show air under the diaphragm in some 70 per cent of patients. As little as 20 ml of free air in the peritoneal cavity will produce the characteristic crescent-shaped shadow between diaphragm and liver. In the remainder of these patients the intake of alcohol has produced an acute gastritis, but there has been no perforation. The pain may be so severe as to be confused with a myo-cardial infarction. If there has been a leak of duodenal contents this may irritate the left leaf of the diaphragm and produce pain behind the left shoulder which can further confuse the diagnosis. An ECG should be performed but its interpretation may be equivocal.

HAEMATEMESIS AND MELAENA

The clinical symptoms of acute gastro-intestinal bleeding are that a patient begins to feel unwell, becomes nauseated, starts to sweat and looks pale. Then, after a variable period of time from minutes to a few hours, the patients vomits up either fresh blood or coffee ground material. Subsequently he may pass a large, soft, tarry, melaena stool. In the Emergency Department resuscitation takes precedence over any effort to determine the site of the bleeding. An intravenous line must be established. Even if the patient is not shocked at this stage he may be-come so. The fluid infused will be determined by the general condition of the patient. Saline may suffice in the mild case, but plasma expander should be used in the more severe case while cross-matched blood is awaited. Occasionally, in the most severe cases, Group O negative blood may have to be used until cross-matched blood becomes available. In recent years the improvement in skills and equipment for fibre optic gastro-enteroscopy has considerably improved the prognosis in the management of these patients.

ACUTE CHOLECYSTITIS

Traditionally it is taught that patients with cholecystitis are fair, fat, forty and female. Some may be, but our studies show that, although the condition is unusual under 40 years of age, its incidence increases with age from the middle years of life onwards.

The pain of acute cholecystitis comes on fairly gradually so that most patients have had symptoms for about 48 hours before they come to hospital. During this time they will also have developed anorexia and nausea and may have vomited. They may have a raised temperature and

70 per cent of them will have had previous attacks – although probably not so severe. Nearly all the patients describe the pain as being on the right-hand side of the abdomen and almost half of them accurately localize it in the right upper quadrant. The pain is made worse by deep inspiration and if they also have right shoulder tip pain then the diagnosis is fairly certain. Jaundice is another confirmatory symptom which is present in about a quarter of all cases. On abdominal palpation there is tenderness in the right upper quadrant. Murphy's sign – pain accompanying inspiration on palpation under the right costal margin – is further strong evidence for the diagnosis. A straight X-ray of the abdomen will help to exclude other abdominal crises, such as small bowel obstruction and perforated duodenal ulcer, and may reveal a gall bladder full of stones.

RENAL COLIC

Severe renal colic is unmistakable. The pain is excruciating. The patient looks grey, sweats, and may roll on the floor in agony. The pain radiates from the loin to the pubic region, often to the penis and scrotum in the male or to the labia in the female. No other disease produces these symptoms. There is no abdominal tenderness or rigidity but palpation of the kidney is usually painful. Strangury is also sometimes present. These symptoms are usually due to a renal calculus making its way down the ureter. Sometimes the stone is held up at the pelvic brim and can be demonstrated on a straight X-ray of the abdomen. When the stone completes its journey to the bladder the colic will cease, but these patients merit subsequent investigation of the urinary tract to detect the presence of other stones or other chronic disease.

RUPTURED ECTOPIC GESTATION AND SALPINGITIS

A young woman, who has recently missed a period, is carried into the Emergency Department looking ashen. There has been a sudden onset of abdominal pain and she may have vomited once. The pulse is weak and rapid and the blood pressure is low. There is generalized abdominal tenderness and the abdomen is doughy. She looks and is exsanguinated. She has a ruptured ectopic pregnancy with a massive haemoperitoneum. Although these patients look as though they are about to die they almost always respond favourably to blood transfusion and surgery.

Acute salpingitis, when it occurs, may mimic a less severe form of ruptured ectopic pregnancy. Vaginal examination will reveal a tender swollen fallopian tube. Arrangements should be made for a gynaecologist to undertake the necessary treatment.

.22

Paediatric Emergencies

A very large part of the work of any Accident Department involves the treatment of children. Unfortunately, it is only of recent years that the special needs of children have been recognized and many departments are totally inadequate in respect of facilities for treating these young patients. Ideally, every department should have a waiting area set aside for children and their parents. Such an area (if it is not available, it can be created in part of the waiting room, screened from the main area yet visible from the clinical area) will do much to reduce the tension affecting both the child and the parents. It is important that the area can be supervised by nursing staff; if parents cannot see, or be seen by, nurses, they will not use the facility in case they may be overlooked. It is also important that the necessary priority can be given to children who begin to feel unwell after they have registered in the department.

As far as is practical, waiting should be kept to a minimum. Even if this is not always possible, a sympathetic word from a member of the staff is always appreciated and allows the parent to draw attention to any problems they may have, such as having to collect another child from school.

It is all too easy for the doctor dealing with large numbers of adult patients to forget that children need a different approach. The manner of the nursing staff towards children and their parents should be studied by the doctor, as it has much to offer. When children appear to be 'difficult', the nursing staff are usually able to quieten them fairly easily by using a cheerful, though sympathetic, approach which, while allowing for the age of the child, accepts that the patient is an individual and not a passive object to be treated mechanically with minimal conversation.

After an injury, both child and parent are upset; the parent's anxiety communicates itself to the child, who is already in a strange and frightening situation and, as a result, the nervous child becomes unapproachable, frightened and clings to the mother in distress. A few minutes spent talking to the child will go far to persuading the child to co-operate. Within limits, after reassurance and explanation, accompanied by a parent even young children will co-operate and allow the doctor to undertake procedures such as foreign body removal from the nose with only minimal protest.

As a general principle, every effort should be made to minimize the occasions which produce crying in children. If one child cries, others in the department tend to follow suit, even though they are not being treated in any way. Apart from the noise level, which can be very high if several children are crying at once, it is preferable that children should not be disturbed before they are seen otherwise their management becomes more difficult.

Some children cannot be consoled by any approach and scream whenever an attempt is made to examine or treat them. Frequently this arises from the parent's failing to help or control the child. The only satisfactory way to handle such a child is for a nurse to take over the handling of the child while the parent waits in another room.

Some children, far from being upset by the situation, appear to be thoroughly enjoying themselves. It is possible with these individuals to have a very pleasant conversation, during which the examination can be carried out without distress to either child or parent. Experience gained in handling this type of child can be applied to similar situations in the more nervous individual with a consequential gain in the doctor's efficiency.

Whenever possible, the parent should accompany the child during the treatment, even if this involves suturing under local anaesthesia. The child who is having a general anaesthetic can be accompanied by the mother until the anaesthetic has been induced. Provided the parent is not over-possessive and liable to interfere with the treatment, or extremely nervous and considered to be unsuitable to be present, nothing but good can come from encouraging the parent to comfort the child during the treatment. External wounds can be sutured under local anaesthetic with as much ease as would be found with a general anesthetic, provided the parents have been told beforehand what is going to be done and what attitude they should adopt during the procedure, but they must be told that if at any time they should feel faint they must report this immediately.

Children may require restraint for the purpose of examination and for treatment if the procedure is in any way uncomfortable. Much depends on the approach of the doctor and the help given by the parents and nursing staff. For example, it is usually an easy matter to inspect the ear drums of children of any age, but the removal of a foreign body from the nose may be dificult because the child keeps withdrawing or moving his head. A small child should be wrapped in a blanket while he is gently laid on a firm examination couch. The pillow should be removed and the head gently restrained by a nurse. It is preferable if the mother can hold the child's hand through the blanket.

Larger children should sit on their parent's knees with their feet held between their parent's thighs. One of the parent's hands holds the child round the chest, trapping his arms, and the other hand holds the child round the forehead in the required position.

If the child is uncontrollable, and the parents appear to be contributing to the situation, it is preferable to separate the child and the parents until the procedures have been completed. Alternatively, if a general anaesthetic will not be required and delay will not be prejudicial, the child can be given an oral dose of 5–20 mg diazepam syrup.

A good general principle in the department is always to question the reason why children should be crying. It is not possible to avoid some children showing distress, but proper handling, together with the use of suitable sedatives and local or general anaesthesia when appropriate, will do much to avoid the development of a fear of doctors and hospitals in the patient.

THE INJURED CHILD

Treatment of the injuries follows the standard principles used in adults, but the junior doctor should be aware of certain important differences which modify the management of the young patient:

1. Certain procedures require the administration of a general anaesthetic. This should always be used if the child is distressed or co-operation cannot be anticipated. Such procedures as the removal of a foreign body from the eye, ear or nose may require this approach and it is always preferable to administer a general anaesthetic rather than causing great distress to the patient. Intravenous anaesthetic agents, used for induction by an anaesthetist skilled in handling children, are painless, rapid in action and free from mental distress. A child who is pale, apprehensive and distressed before the procedure usually looks significantly improved on recovery from the anaesthetic.

2. Children tend to 'over-react' to illness or injury when compared to adults suffering from similar conditions. For example, children after head injuries frequently present in the department with pallor which is out of proportion to the degree of the injury. It is a safe assumption to make that any child showing such pallor will vomit profusely within a very short time. After vomiting and a short rest, the child appears completely recovered. Management depends on the overall assessment of the head injury.

   Similarly, children are very prone to develop convulsions after head injury. This apparently serious complication must be treated by intravenous use of an anti-convulsant drug, e.g. 2–10 mg diazepam followed by admission for observation. The prognosis is good in these cases and complications are unlikely to follow.

Similar pallor is found in children who swallow blood from epistaxis or a bleeding tooth socket. Provided the blood loss is relatively small and insufficient to affect the haemodynamic response, vomiting is a likely occurrence.

3. Children react very quickly to blood loss, whether from open wounds or concealed haemorrhage. It is important to realize that it is the percentage of the circulating blood and not the absolute amount lost that is significant. An adult can easily lose 500 ml from the circulation without any adverse effect, but a similar sized haemorrhage in a child with a blood volume of only 2 litres would show significant effects and require urgent replacement therapy. Therefore all haemorrhage from wounds, and particularly those of the scalp and face, should be dealt with expeditiously and the bleeding controlled by pressure, ligature or suture, depending on the circumstances.

When external haemorrhage from, for example, a wound or a tooth socket, does not stop with the appropriate measures, the possibility of a bleeding diathesis must be considered, and it may be necessary to seek the advice of the Paediatric Unit, who should also be asked for assistance if difficulties are encountered in setting up an intravenous drip on a very small child.

Concern over the physical well-being of the child should not blind the doctor to the importance of determining the cause of the accident. The prevention of accidents is an important part of the work of any unit and, without information about the causation, prevention is not possible. Even without an organized information retrieval system, the individual doctor should be able to spot situations which need correction if further incidents are to be avoided. This is primarily a matter of taking the history a little deeper than might be considered appropriate in an older person. For example, if a child falls out of a window, the reason why he or she fell out should be established. It could be that he was pushed out by another child – this would call for an investigation into the family dynamics in case there was great jealousy for the younger child by an older child. Alternatively, there might be no safety devices on the window to prevent it opening enough to allow the child to fall through. The sill might be too low; a feature of this nature might be found in many houses on an estate and all the children would be at risk.

When several children are injured under similar circumstances in the same area, the hazard is more obvious but, even in isolated cases, it is frequently possible to find situations which present a danger to children and for which suggestions for correction can be made to the parents. Such suggestions should be made in a sympathetic manner. The parents of a child who has been injured by a situation which should have been corrected or which, on hind-sight, can be seen to be dangerous, may well have a feeling of guilt. Time should be taken to reassure them, using a non-accusatory manner. The Medical Social Worker can supplement this advice or help by a home visit; alternatively, the Health Visiting Services could be asked to call. Health Visitors have an important part to play in accident prevention in children; they have a statutory duty to care for children under five. Their acceptance by the parents enables them to visit the home after injury and, apart from giving relevant advice about the care of the child, allows accident prevention to be discussed in home surroundings.

It is easier to deal with accident prevention in the home when only one family is involved. Hazardous situations in schools, playgroups or other public places require the involvement of the local authorities and are referred preferably to the consultant in charge of the department for him to take up the matter with the appropriate branch of the local authority.

Few situations cause such distress in a department as the arrival of a seriously ill or dead child after an accident. Many of the points mentioned later under 'Cot deaths' are relevant to the care of the parents of these children. The degree of parental distress can be extreme and sedation may be required. Diazepam (10–30 mg) is helpful under these circumstances, but the greatest help is obtained by sending for the other parent or a near relative. The general practitioner can be asked to call on the family when the parents have returned home and, if necessary, the Medical Social Worker will be able to involve the Social Services Department if it appears that the incident will add further problems to a family already suffering from significant social disruption.

An adult who seriously injures or kills a child accidentally will be subjected to major stress, associated with strong feelings of guilt. This must not be overlooked in the desire to give attention to the child and his parents. Reassurance, explanation, sedation and the involvement of the general practitioner may be equally necessary, but it is important, from a legal point of view, that the person who caused the injury should be advised that, irrespective of his feelings or the cause of the accident, he should never indicate to the parents that the accident was his fault. To do so would prejudice any action that might be considered appropriate by his insurance company and might be used in a prosecution against him. Even though it may appear unsympathetic and go against everyone's natural inclination, it is preferable that the two groups be kept apart and conversation between them limited to the absolute minimum.

COT DEATHS

Sudden death in infancy resulting from as yet inadequately understood causes results in the death of about 2000 children under the age of 2, annually. The child, who appears perfectly healthy, is found dead in his cot a few minutes or hours after he was put to bed. Vomit or blood-stained fluid may be found in the mouth or on the bedding, but is minimal and not the cause of death. At *post mortem* it is unusual to find any significant disease except unsuspected congenital abnormalities or rapidly progressive infections, such as pneumonia or meningitis. The disorder can occur in children of all social classes but is commoner in the more deprived section of the community.

The parents develop strong guilt feelings and devote much time to considering whether they were in any way to blame and whether they might have prevented the child's death. It is more important to explain to them that the condition is well recognized but ill-understood and that no blame is attached to anyone.

Even if the child appears to be dead in the ambulance, it is advisable to take him into the department. An adequate examination can be carried out, death from obvious violence can be excluded and resuscitation, even though unsuccessful, will reassure the parents that everything that could be done has been done. Resuscitation is primarily a matter of clearing the upper airway using suction, the use of a small manual ventilator to ventilate the lungs with oxygen and external cardiac massage if the heart has stopped. In a small child, one or two fingers may be used to apply the necessary pressure to the sternum. Excessive force may cause serious damage to the abdominal or thoracic viscera.

Another member of the staff should obtain the history during the attempt at resuscitation but, when death is established, the doctor, accompanied by a trained nurse, should see the parents. It should be explained to them that death appears to be a 'cot death', that this condition is not well understood and that the coroner will have to be informed. He will order a *post mortem* examination, but an inquest is not a necessary sequel, nor is it likely that anyone will be blamed for the occurrence. The parents should be given the opportunity to see the child's body if they desire and they should be asked if they wish a minister of religion to attend.

The Coroner's Officer must be informed and the Social Services or Health Visitor should also be notified if they are involved with the family. It is important that the family doctor be notified; he may consider it necessary to visit the family at home and later arrange to discuss the *post mortem* results with them. Alternatively, some paediatricians with an interest in the disease are prepared, with the consent of the practitioner, to discuss the whole situation with the parents in an attempt to provide support in a situation of considerable emotional strain. This stress may also affect the more junior members of the department, particularly the nurses, and they should be given the opportunity to talk the matter through with their seniors.

NON-ACCIDENTAL INJURIES

This widely publicized condition is relatively infrequent in a busy department. Nevertheless, because it has a high mortality and morbidity and is responsible for much suffering, an awareness of the disorder is essential among doctors who work in Accident and Emergency Departments.

In one department treating 40 000 patients every year, 40 cases of non-accidental injury may possibly be seen. It is therefore a relatively small problem in relation to the total workload of the department, but this should not obscure the importance of the early recognition of the condition. The disorder has an appreciable death rate, a considerable morbidity and emotional effects which may affect the child for the rest of his life. If the condition is recognized in good time, steps can be taken to correct the disturbances in the family unit, which are the primary causes of the disease and, in the majority of cases, a successful outcome can be anticipated.

It is important to realize that the child's parents are in need of help and should not be treated by any members of the staff in a manner other than that used for other patients. The approach should be non-accusatory and expressions of disapproval and criticism must be avoided. Treatment will be carried out by the paediatric services, working in conjunction with the social and other services and any exhibition of hostility in the initial contacts will make case work in the future very much more difficult or even impossible.

The situation must be kept in perspective. An enthusiasm to contain the disorder must not lead to a witch hunt. By far the largest number of children attending a department are suffering from accidents, and it would be completely unjustified for the parents of these children to feel that they were in any way under suspicion. The diagnosis depends on a combination of the medical findings considered together with the clinical aspects of the case. Suspicion is raised by the history, in which there are certain alerting features:

1. There is delay in seeking treatment for a condition for which a parent would normally seek immediate advice. This may vary from an hour or two to a week or longer.
2. The younger the child, the more it is important to establish the precise and detailed cause of the injury.

3. The history may appear superficially reasonable but, on detailed enquiry, can be seen to be inappropriate for the injury.
4. The history is completely incompatible with the injury.
5. There are significant differences in the history given by the parents to each person who takes the history.
6. If the child is alleged to be responsible for causing his own injuries, his physical development must be compatible with the mechanism of the injury.
7. The parents, who are receiving support from the community services, fail to bring the child to hospital until they are brought to the department by a member of the service. There may be a genuine reason for this happening, e.g. a large family with several young members, and it is advisable to discuss this with the person who brings the child to hospital.

Concern should also be felt for children who are repeatedly seen in the department with injuries. All children sustain injuries, but the repeat attender may well be living under circumstances which are in need of correction.

Examination must be thorough and the whole body should be inspected in a good light. A record is made of the child's development, clothing and response to the staff of the department. A detailed record is made of each individual lesion on the skin.

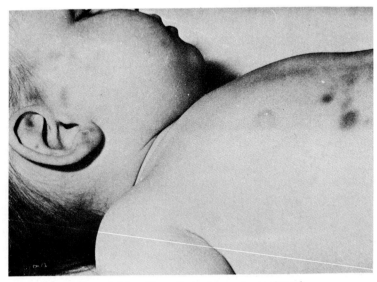

Figure 22.1. Finger tip bruises on face and trunk

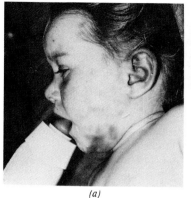
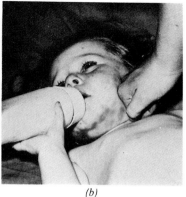

(a)   *(b)*

Figure 22.2. (a) Finger tip bruising on face associated with a 'purple ear'. Linear bruising is also visible on the left cheek. (b) The linear bruising matched with great accuracy a closed fist, which was also responsible for the injury to the ear

Finger tip bruises occur in groups, which may be of different ages and vary in size between 4–20 mm in diameter. They are found in all areas of the body *(Figure 22.1)* and, when they are present on the face, the condition can be recognized from some distance away *(Figure 22.2)*. Slap marks from the flat of the hand or a slipper are common and frequently two or more types can be found on the same child *(Figure 22.3)*. The frenulum of the upper lip may be torn and the lip bruised from a blow. The inner aspect of the lip may be lacerated against the edge of a tooth *(Figure 22.4)*.

Haemorrhage may be present in the tympanic membrane when the ear has been hit. Conjunctival haemorrhage may be present in other cases and retinal haemorrhage or other ocular damage may be found after blows or in association with subdural haemorrhage.

Black eyes are of considerable significance. It is physically impossible to injure both eyes in the same fall and such lesions in very young children are almost pathognomonic of the condition *(Figure 22.5)*.

Subdural haemorrhage is usually caused by shaking and, in some cases, symmetrical paired bruises can be found, indicating that the child has been held in a manner compatible with forcible shaking. These bruises have been seen on each side, about 6 cm from the midline opposite the 12th dorsal or 1st lumbar vertebra, in the middle of the inner aspect of each upper arm, over the front of each shoulder and on each ear *(Figure 22.6)*.

Other lesions seen include blows from straps, loops of rope or slippers, bites *(Figure 22.7)*, pinches, burns *(Figures 22.8 and 22.9)* and scalds and cigarette burns *(Figure 22.10)*.

226

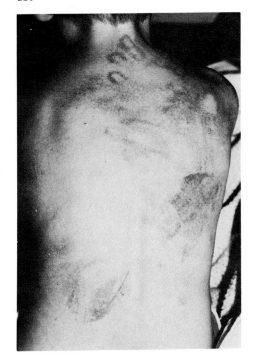

Figure 22.3. Imprints of a hand and the heel and sole of a slipper on a child's back

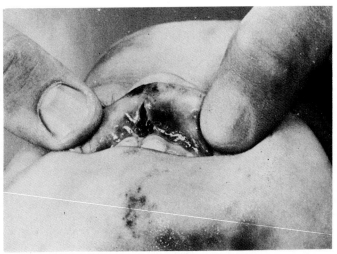

Figure 22.4. Bruising and a torn frenulum of the upper lip due to a blow

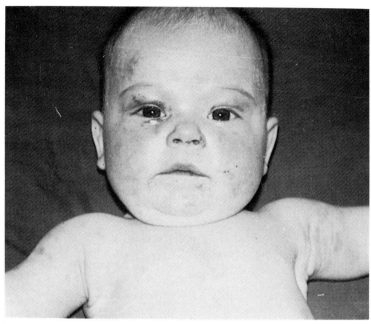

Figure 22.5. Bruising of both eyelids on the right side and the upper eyelids on the left side. This child also exhibited finger tip bruising of the right forehead and right upper arm

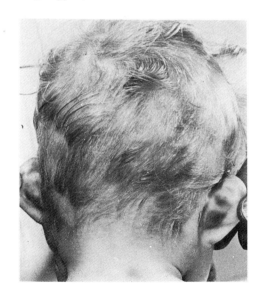

Figure 22.6. Finger tip bruising of both ears; this child died from a bilateral subdural haemorrhage caused by shaking

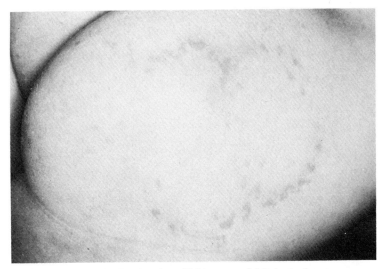

Figure 22.7. Imprint of 3 bites on a child's buttocks

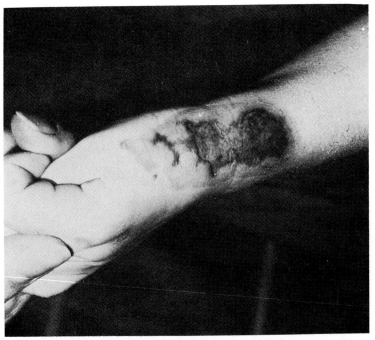

Figure 22.8. Full thickness burn caused by an electric iron

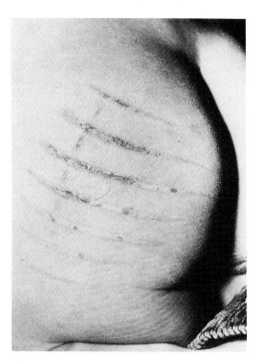

Figure 22.9. Burns of buttock caused by holding against wire guard on electric fire

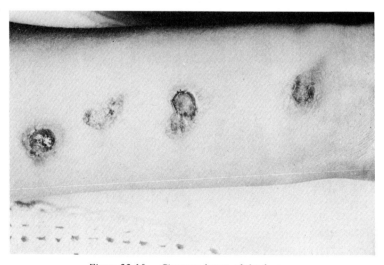

Figure 22.10. Cigarette burns of the forearm

Major intra-abdominal lesions may be present without external bruising. These have a high mortality and treatment must take precedence over any social investigation that may be felt necessary.

The limbs and trunk should be palpated for evidence of bony damage and a skeletal survey should be carried out in most cases. The X-rays will reveal recent fractures and deformity or callus formation from previous bony injuries.

Burns and scalds present major difficulties and recognition that they are of a non-accidental causation depends on incongruities between the history and the distribution of the lesion. Occasionally, as after burns from electric irons or cooker rings, the shape is diagnostic but, in the majority of the cases, all that the doctor may acquire is a strong feeling of unease which cannot be quantified.

If the history and examination suggest that there is a possibility that the child might have sustained a non-accidental injury, the child should be referred to the Paediatric Department for further investigation, treatment and protection.

It must not be forgotten that certain injuries may have been inflicted by other children in the family. Typical sibling injuries include hair pulling, leaving small bare areas of the scalp, pinches, bites and blows with various objects.

The differential diagnosis includes 'true' accidents, fragilitas ossium, giving rise to repeated fractures, purpura, simulating finger tip bruising, bony tumours, simulating callus formation and mongoloid spots. This latter condition, found in pigmented races, is characterized by blue-coloured pigmented areas, typically in the skin of the lower back and sacrum. Smaller, discrete areas may closely simulate finger tip bruising and, with an increasing number of children from immigrant families in the population, the condition must not be overlooked.

All districts now have their own routine for the management of non-accidental injuries, which should be followed whenever a suspected case is seen. If the junior doctor is uncertain about his diagnosis and the appropriate action to take, this should be discussed with his consultant or a senior member of the Paediatric Department. Delay in initiating treatment can have serious consequences for the child, whose well-being must be given high priority using, if necessary, admission in order to remove him from the hazards of his home surroundings.

FOREIGN BODIES

The diagnosis of a 'foreign body' is usually straightforward when the area can be inspected directly. Similarly, radio-opaque objects do not present difficulties in confirmation, but many are either completely or partially radio-lucent. When X-raying to demonstrate a foreign body, the nature of the object should be stated on the X-ray request form. If the foreign body is thought to be unlikely to show clearly on the X-ray film, it may be helpful to X-ray a similar foreign body on a comparable part of the patient's body. This may enable objects which would not otherwise be demonstrable on the film, because of soft tissue shadows, to be identified with a reasonable degree of certainty.

Foreign bodies in the eye

It may be possible to remove a foreign body from the eye using local anaesthetic and a cotton wool pledget on an orange stick. The child should be lying on a firm surface and wrapped in a blanket to prevent movement. If the foreign body is firmly embedded in the cornea, it is unlikely that it will be possible to remove it except with a needle and the assistance of the Eye Department should be obtained.

Foreign bodies in the nose

Foreign bodies in the nose can usually be removed using topical anaesthesia. The child should be on a firm surface and wrapped in a blanket. Occasionally the foreign body can be gripped in forceps but firm, round objects, e.g. beads, cannot be gripped with nasal forceps. The forceps slip off the object and may drive it further back into the nasal passages. They must be removed by applying pressure from behind and pulling the object forwards. A curved dissector or a probe with the tip bent over is a suitable instrument for the purpose. If the object is situated well back and high up in the nose, the ENT Department should be consulted. If it cannot be removed easily or bleeding starts, referral is indicated. Indeed it is always wise to stop before bleeding is started by unskilled attempts at removal. Bleeding makes the task of the surgeon much more difficult and it is an axiom of work in the Accident and Emergency Department that the task of any doctor taking over a case from the unit shall not be made more difficult by unskilled or inappropriate management in the department.

If the foreign body has been in the nose for several days, it will be partly obscured by swelling of the tissues and a discharge, which is usually foul smelling. Peanuts may become very firmly impacted because they swell in the presence of moisture from the nasal secretions.

Foreign bodies in the ear

Foreign bodies in the external auditory meatus are technically difficult to remove because of the necessity to work through a speculum, using special instruments. The majority of children with these foreign bodies should be referred to the ENT Department rather than cause damage from unskilled attempts at removal. Syringing is not usually advisable. If the meatus is completely occluded, this would force the foreign body further in and might damage the drum. It is contra-indicated in the presence of a perforation and further damage could be caused by movement of the child during the procedure. It should only be attempted with foreign bodies which are superficial and do not occlude the meatus. Minimal pressure is essential and the jet of water should be directed towards the gap above or at the side of the foreign body. The position of the foreign body must be checked frequently and the attempt stopped if it does not move. If the attempt is successful the meatus should be gently dried with cotton wool pledgets and the drum inspected to exclude damage.

Inhaled foreign bodies

Inhaled foreign bodies are associated with an attack of coughing and respiratory distress of a varying degree. If the distress persists, it suggests some degree of occlusion of the air passages.

The pharynx should be inspected with the child in the head-down position. If the foreign body can be seen to be near the larynx, removal should only be attempted if suitable instruments are available. If the foreign body becomes dislodged and occludes the larynx, the child should promptly be held in the air by the feet and the back smacked. The urgency of the situation is such that manual removal or dislodgment with a finger should be tried, otherwise tracheostomy may be required. This is technically very difficult in a young child with respiratory occlusion and it is advisable to avoid attempting any procedure which may result in this being necessary.

If it is thought that the object has entered one of the bronchi, an X-ray should be taken. Radio-opaque foreign bodies are clearly demonstrated but, unfortunately, many objects do not show directly on the film and their presence may have to be deduced by the development of changes in the lungs. If there is a strong probability of an inhaled foreign body being present based on the history and possibly on the presence of abnormalities in the breath sounds, the child should be referred to the ENT Department with a view to bronchoscopy.

When there is a possibility of a radio-lucent foreign body, the chest should be re-X-rayed after 4 hours. Occlusion of a bronchus will produce collapse of the appropriate segment of the lungs.

No child should be discharged from medical supervision until the doctor is satisfied that the foreign body is not in the lungs. This may require further X-rays at weekly intervals until the absence of pulmonary changes confirms the absence of the foreign body, and it is always advisable to notify the general practitioner about the situation in case chest symptoms arise in the more remote future and the possibility of a foreign body may be overlooked if the information is not available.

All cases must be dealt with on their merits and, while most alleged inhaled foreign bodies have either been swallowed or coughed out, it is unsafe to assume that this has occurred without taking steps to ensure that a negative initial assessment will not prejudice the child's future well-being.

Foreign bodies in the oesophagus

Foreign bodies impacted in the oesophagus give rise to difficulty in swallowing. Radio-lucent foreign bodies cannot be seen on X-ray, but should be suspected if the child is unable to swallow water. The presence of such a foreign body can be confirmed by a barium swallow, using a minimal amount of contrast medium, but if the child is considered to need a contrast medium investigation, it is preferable to refer him to the ENT Department without further investigation.

Swallowed foreign bodies

Swallowed foreign bodies smaller in diameter than a 5p piece (23mm) should pass through any child old enough to swallow such an object. If it can be clearly established that the foreign body is of such a size that it will pass through the child, there is little point in X-ray examination. The parents should be advised to allow the child a normal diet and not administer purgatives. The motions should be examined under water to see if the foreign body has been passed. Unless the child develops symtoms such as abdominal pain or vomiting, concern need not be felt if the foreign body is not found.

X-Ray examination is advisable to detect the presence of sharp metallic objects, such as a pin, an open safety pin or a nail, or objects which might not pass through because of their size or shape. When X-ray shows a pin or similar pointed object, the child should be admitted in case the foreign body perforates the intestine. Objects which might not pass through should have their progress studied in serial X-rays at daily or longer intervals until they have been excreted. If they do not progress through the alimentary tract, the child should be referred to the Surgical Unit in case laparotomy is necessary. The parents must be advised, if the child is being treated as an out-patient, to bring him or her back to the department immediately if abdominal pain or vomiting develops.

POISONING

A safe assumption, when dealing with children, is that there is no solid or liquid substance which has properties that will inhibit a child from attempting to eat or drink it. Fortunately, in spite of their catholic tastes in this direction, the annual mortality remains low, but the number of children admitted to hospital for treatment or, more usually, for observation remains high. Household cleaning products are high on the list of substances, but drugs and medicines prescribed for the child, the parents, the grandparents or neighbours are one of the groups that cause concern. The other group of dangerous products is garden chemicals. These, for example paraquat, are highly toxic.

The Accident Officer should always be aware of his responsibility in the field of accident prevention by finding out how the child obtained the substance which has brought him to hospital and, if appropriate, make suggestions to the parents to avoid the situation recurring. The parents are frequently distressed after poisoning incidents and, if it is felt inappropriate at that time, the Health Visitor can be asked to make a home visit at a later date when advice may be more acceptable.

Management

The management of a case of poisoning in the Emergency Department involves:

1. The identification of the poison.
2. The treatment of any serious effects, e.g. convulsions or respiratory paralysis.
3. The elimination of the poison.
4. Admission to the Paediatric Department.

Identification of the poison

Identification may sometimes be a matter of informed guesswork, but usually the parents are sensible enough to bring a sample of the container to the hospital. Suitable tablet identification charts and reference books, which should be available in every department, are consulted to identify the precise nature of the chemical component, the specific treatment that may be needed and the various toxic effects that may arise. Reference can also be made to one of the Poisons Centres (*see* Appendix I) which hold comprehensive information about all the various aspects of drugs, chemicals and other products that are found within the home and in industry.

Estimation of the amount that the child may have consumed is also difficult. The majority of children spit the substance out without swallowing more than an insignificant amount but, when there is any possibility of a clinically significant consumption, a blood estimation should be carried out or, if appropriate, the laboratory should be asked to do a rapid screening test for some of the commoner drugs that are likely to be available to the child.

Blood estimations should always be carried out after the consumption of aspirin, barbiturates, psychotropic drugs, ferrous sulphate, paraquat and alcohol. Alcohol may produce significant hypoglycaemia and a blood sugar estimation should be done at the same time.

The time of consumption is important in relation to the development of symptoms and the necessity to carry out active treatment.

Initial treatment

Major adverse effects should be treated immediately. Respiratory depression takes precedence over all other aspects of the situation. The pharynx should be cleared by suction and an airway inserted, after which the child should be placed in the recovery position. Oxygen should be given through a face mask and, if these measures prove insufficient, assisted ventilation, using an Ambu bag or similar apparatus should be commenced. This can be followed by intubation and mechanical ventilation if the child does not make a very rapid improvement.

Convulsions should be controlled by intravenous diazepam: 0.25 mg per kilo of body weight, up to 1 year of age; 2.5 mg between 1 and 7 years of age; 5 mg over 7 years of age.

Circulatory collapse with a systolic blood pressure below 100 mmHg should be treated with an intravenous infusion of normal glocose or normal glucose with $^1/_5$ normal saline. Normal saline should not be used to avoid salt retention caused by overloading the child's kidney with NaCl.

The Paediatric Department should always be consulted at an early stage when signs of toxicity are apparent, but urgent treatment must not be delayed while waiting for the arrival of either the paediatric or anaesthetic services.

Elimination of the poison

Most swallowed poisons are best treated by inducing vomiting with syrup of ipecacuanha: 10 ml from 6 to 18 months, and 15 ml if older. Half to one cup of water (or orange juice) should be given with the emetic. If vomiting does not occur within 20 minutes, the dose should be repeated.

If vomiting does still not occur, it is essential that the stomach should be washed out to remove the emetic. The emetic should not be used if the patient is other than fully conscious, nor should vomiting be induced in kerosene or petrol poisoning because these substances are of greater danger if they contaminate the lungs than if they are left in the stomach.

Strong salt solutions are dangerous to use as emetics because of the risk of biochemical disturbances developing from the absorption of the sodium chloride.

Most drugs are absorbed or leave the stomach within 2 to 3 hours and there is little point in inducing vomiting after this time. Aspirin and ferrous sulphate are unusual because significant quantities can be recovered even after periods of 6 to 8 hours and it is well worthwhile to induce vomiting even after this time.

Tricyclic antidepressants rapidly cause ileus and may be recovered after many hours, but they should be removed by gastric lavage as ipecacuanha is unlikely to work.

When removal of the drug is considered essential and the patient is unconscious, the air passages should be protected by a cuffed endotracheal tube before lavage is commenced. Water is an effective solution to use for this purpose and the procedure should be continued until the returns are clear. The head-down position must be used and every care taken to safeguard the respiratory tract. The mouth should be sucked clear at the end of the procedure and, if there is any doubt about the ability of the child to maintain a clear airway, the tube should be left in place.

The stomach contents should be preserved for laboratory investigation if the child presents the slightest sign of toxic effects or if the substance consumed cannot be identified.

Admission

Admission should always follow treatment in the Emergency Department. In most cases the child will not show any ill-effects from the drug or chemical and observation for longer than 6 to 8 hours will not be necessary. The parents should be informed about the child's condition and the reason for admission, but it should be made clear that the responsibility for treatment has been handed over to the paediatric service.

Some specific poisons

Aspirin poisoning

Confirmation that the child has taken this drug can be obtained by the use of 'phenistix', which turns a deep purple colour when dipped in the child's urine.

Blood levels should be ascertained if the child is vomiting or hyper-ventilating. The drug produces a metabolic acidosis with a respiratory alkalosis, and blood gas and pH estimations are necessary for treatment after the stomach contents have been removed. Treatment is carried out by the Paediatric Department.

Ferrous sulphate

This highly toxic drug is frequently taken by children who swallow tablets that have been prescribed for their mothers and which have been left lying around the home. Vomiting is an early symptom. Gastric erosions may cause haematemesis and shock. Prompt treatment is essential. Vomiting should be induced with ipecacuanha and the stomach should then be washed out using 2 g desferrioxamine in 1 litre of water; 10 g desferrioxamine in 50 ml of water should be left in the stomach and absorbed iron can be treated by an intramuscular injection of 1–2 g desferrioxamine in 5–10 ml of water.

A blood sample should be sent to the laboratory to provide a primary level of the free iron content of the plasma.

Paraquat

This substance and the closely related substances diquat and granmoxone are usually consumed by accident from the habit of gardeners and farmers leaving the solution in lemonade or similar bottles around the premises.

The substance is inactivated by contact with soil and, as a First Aid measure, a tablespoon of soil mixed in a cup of water should be given to the child. Vomiting should be induced by pharyngeal stimulation.

In hospital the stomach should be washed out with water.

Even small amounts can be fatal and, as the onset of symptoms may be delayed for 2 or 3 days, admission is imperative.

Confirmation of consumption can be obtained from urine examin-ation. Further treatment is carried out as an in-patient and the parents should be warned that the child may become very seriously ill.

Paracetamol

Ipecacuanha should be used to produce vomiting. A blood level esti-mation should be carried out.

Treatment with cysteamine should be left to the paediatricians to carry out, but good results (Solomon, A. E., Briggs, J. D., Knepil, I, Henry, D. A., Winchester, J. F. and Birrell, R. 1977. 'Therapeutic comparison of thiol compounds in severe paracetamol poisoning'. *Ann.*

clin. Biochem., **14**, 200) have been obtained from the early use of intravenous amino-acid solutions which contain this substance, commenced as soon as initial treatment has been concluded. Suitable solutions are those used for intravenous nutrition and they should be given at a rate appropriate to the size of the child.

Barbiturates

If the child is fully conscious, vomiting should be induced with ipecacuanha. The blood level and type of barbiturate should be established, because the patient's response varies greatly with the drug, being more marked with short-acting rather than long-acting barbiturates in equivalent doses.

When the respiratory depression has progressed to complete paralysis, intubation and mechanical ventilation are essential. This will also be essential if the child is cyanosed. Lesser degrees of depression may require the administration of oxygen through a face mask, but it is important to realize that hypoxia can be present even in the absence of cyanosis.

Blood gas analysis may be necessary and assistance from the Anaesthetic Department should be sought if the depth and rate of respiration appear to be diminished.

When the child is unconscious, gastric lavage should be carried out if the drug was consumed less than 2 hours before admission and the airway has been protected by a cuffed endotracheal tube. It must never be undertaken on any patient who is unable to protect his own airway without intubation having been carried out first. Provided hypoxia and circulatory collapse are controlled, the results are good and the use of analeptics or other stimulants is neither advisable nor necessary.

The phenothiazines and tricyclic antidepressants

Large amounts of these drugs are in use among the population and consumption of a parent's capsules is not infrequent. The former are less toxic than the latter, but they can both cause disturbances of consciousness and respiratory depression.

Treatment follows standard practice but it should be noted that both can give rise to cardiac arrhythmias. The patients should be carefully monitored on a cardioscope and the Paediatric Department contacted immediately if arrhythmias appear. Admission is essential, even if the amount consumed appears to be minimal.

Household products, cosmetics, etc.

There are vast numbers of proprietary products found in every house, garage, greenhouse or other outbuilding. These may include industrial products brought home by a parent for a particular purpose, e.g. dry cleaning clothes. They may contain petroleum products, corrosives and various complex and possibly toxic chemicals. Respiratory and circulatory depression should be treated immediately, but no attempt to induce vomiting or wash out the stomach should be made until the nature of the substances consumed has been established. The poisons information centres have been provided with details of the formulation of most of the commoner proprietary preparations (e.g. metal cleaners, paints, polishes, etc.) on a confidential basis for use in treating patients, and they should be consulted whenever there is doubt about either the nature of the substance or the treatment necessary. Help may also be obtained locally from schools, colleges or firms in the neighbourhood and from time to time it may be necessary to consult the manufacturers of the particular product. The fire brigade also keeps a comprehensive index of industrial chemicals which are transported by road or which can be produced in fires, and the local College of Agriculture may be of assistance in the identification of plants, seeds or other vegetable products.

MEDICAL EMERGENCIES

Convulsions

One of the commonest paediatric emergencies is a young child suffering from convulsions. He is usually brought in at high speed by a very distressed mother. It is important to find out if the child has suffered from fits or black-outs, if he or she is receiving any medication and if there is a history of an injury or a febrile or other illness during the previous few days.

The convulsions must be controlled immediately. Up to 10 mg diazepam (depending on the child's age) should be given slowly intravenously. An airway is inserted, the pharynx cleared with a sucker and the child nursed in the recovery position.

The Paediatric Department should be notified of any case of convulsions in the Emergency Department, as the child will require admission. If the convulsions do not cease within 15 minutes, the Anaesthetic Department should be consulted because of the risk to the child of asphyxia, inhalation of vomit, permanent neurological deficiencies or even death. Status epilepticus, the condition in which the convulsions do not cease spontaneously or following treatment, may necessitate the induction of general anaesthesia and the use of muscle relaxants to enable a mechanical ventilator to be used until the fits have been brought under control.

The commonest cause of convulsions in children under the age of 5 years is a fever. Certain children, and often siblings, appear to have a genetic predisposition to react in this way. The cause of the fever may be an upper respiratory infection or, in many cases, this condition has left the child with a middle ear infection which can be recognized through an auriscope. Apart from the use of anticonvulsive drugs, the child's temperature should be lowered by exposure and tepid sponging.

Fits may recur in the future if the child suffers a febrile illness, and it may be advisable to administer anticonvulsants on these occasions.

The parents should be reassured that one or two attacks of this nature are not due to epilepsy and that this response to a raised body temperature will probably cease by the time the child is 5 or 6 years of age.

Respiratory emergencies

Respiratory emergencies are properly the responsibility of the paediatric services. However, from time to time children are admitted with acute respiratory embarrassment which demands immediate attention from the Accident Officer. The principal conditions under this heading are status asthmaticus and croup.

Status asthmaticus

Status asthmaticus may develop suddenly during the night in an asthmatic child who has developed a minor upper respiratory infection. The clinical picture is one of marked cyanosis, over-action of the accessory muscles of respiration, retraction of the sternum and intercostal spaces, and obvious great distress in the child. The parents are very upset and the nursing staff are deeply concerned. The doctor should, if necessary, try and reduce the tension by reassuring the child and the parents.

Oxygen should be administered — if this can be given through an efficient humidifier it will be of greater benefit.

Aminophylline (40—100 mg, depending on the age) should be given very slowly intravenously; if it is given too rapidly, there is a danger of cardiac irregularities developing. If this does not result in improvement, intravenous hydrocortisone should be given in a dose of 100 mg. There is no risk of steroid therapy used in the short term producing any of the adverse effects seen when it is used for long-term treatment.

If the child still fails to improve, intermittent positive-pressure ventilation, using a high pressure, to overcome the bronchial spasm may be required. This treatment will be given by the Anaesthetic Department after consultation with the paediatricians.

Croup

Croup is the term commonly applied to a mixed group of conditions in which there is marked respiratory dysfunction which may kill the child if immediate steps are not taken to improve the airway. The conditions, except for an unsuspected inhaled foreign body, are all infective in origin.

Spasmodic croup.   Spasmodic croup commences with an upper respiratory infection in which there is a spread of infection causing congestion and swelling of the vocal cords. The clinical picture of cyanosis, inspiratory stridor and respiratory distress is caused by spasm of the larynx which commonly lasts up to 4 hours, after which the child appears to recover. If, in spite of humidification and sedation the spasm does not wear off after a few hours, intubation should be performed, especially if the cyanosis and respiratory embarrassment do not resolve. Children in this condition may suddenly collapse and develop acute cardiac failure. Therefore all cases of laryngitis should be referred to the paediatricians, even if the child does not appear to be ill.

Acute epiglottitis

This is an acute inflammatory oedema of the larynx. It is usually seen in children between the ages of 2 and 7 years and is caused by an *H. influenzae* infection. Fortunately it is uncommon because the child can be seen to be seriously ill and intubation, which is the appropriate treatment, is technically extremely difficult, even to those posessing the necessary skills.

The condition starts after a minor upper respiratory infection, which is followed by a progressive stridor. There is marked cyanosis and overaction of the inspiratory muscles. The child is quiet, frightened and possibly semi-conscious.

An attempt at intubation may precipitate acute respiratory obstruction. The necessary equipment for tracheostomy must be available before starting to pass an endotracheal tube.

On inspection, the larynx is grossly swollen, the vocal cords being difficult to distinguish because of the oedema. It may not be possible to identify the gap between the cords with clarity and, because of this, every effort should be made to obtain the services of a skilled anaesthetist. The Accident Officer should only attempt the procedure if such help is not available. Tracheostomy, which is not to be undertaken except as a last resort, is extremely hazardous unless expert help is available.

Ampicillin is the antibiotic of choice and highly humidified oxygen should be given once the respiratory obstruction has been relieved.

Acute laryngotracheobronchitis

This is caused by a virus infection which may have a secondary bacterial infection superimposed.

The disease in its late, and dangerous, form presents with toxaemia, oedema of the larynx and thick secretions in the trachea and bronchi which produce respiratory obstruction. The child may be cyanosed and will show over-action of all the respiratory muscles.

Highly humidifed oxygen and tracheal toilet, using a sucker, may prove adequate to relieve the initial acute situation but, if the child's condition deteriorates further, tracheal toilet may be improved by doing this initially under direct vision. Tracheostomy may be necessary to allow adequate tracheal toilet, but it should not be carried out in the Emergency Department.

Gastro-enteritis

It is not uncommon for parents whose children are suffering from gastro-enteritis of infancy to by-pass their general practitioner and bring the child straight to the Emergency Department. The children of caravan dwellers, who have no permanent address and whose hygiene is at best of doubtful quality, are particularly prone to this disorder. Similarly, some immigrant families have strange — by European standards — ideas about infant feeding.

Emergency treatment is unlikely to be needed, but it is important that the child is referred to the paediatricians, even though the doctor may feel aggrieved at being asked to deal with a situation which is not normally regarded as being within the functions of the department. These children can deteriorate very quickly and, if sent home to unsuitable surroundings, it is probable that they will require urgent admission within a short time.

23

Medical Emergencies

The management of a medical emergency arriving unexpectedly in a department fully occupied with the treatment of a large number of traumatic cases presents the inexperienced junior doctor with many problems. In contrast to patients in the out-patient departments, a good history is usually unobtainable. The patient is frightened, distressed, confused or, in many cases, unconscious. It is unusual to obtain a history of previous illnesses or conditions for which the patient is currently being treated by his practitioner and personal information in a handbag or wallet may be insufficient to enable a relative or the patient's practitioner to be contacted.

The Emergency Department has 4 functions in the management of a medical emergency, and it is important that the doctor realizes the limitations imposed on his clinical management because of the circumstances that exist in these units. The doctor should follow a standard routine when dealing with any unexpected medical emergency — he should avoid making 'spot' diagnoses and should try and avoid being rushed into making decisions before he has had time to consider, and if necessary discuss, the appropriate management of the patient. It is easy in a busy atmosphere of an Emergency Department to make errors of judgment. Many such errors do not affect the well-being of the patient in any way, but it is difficult to defend errors such as sending patients home when they live on their own and are not physically fit to care for themselves. A study of the newspaper columns will produce other examples and, if they are to be avoided, the doctor should develop a standard approach which he uses for cases of this nature.

THE MANAGEMENT OF A MEDICAL EMERGENCY

Immediate emergency care

When appropriate, the first step should always be the establishment of a clear airway. Noisy breathing means airway obstruction. This may be caused by the tongue or by vomit or both. The obstruction should be relieved by positioning, the insertion of an airway, clearing the pharynx by suction and, if all else fails, intubation should be carried out and a cuffed endotracheal tube inserted.

Cyanosis will require the administration of oxygen by face mask or through a rebreathing bag connected to an endotracheal tube if the simpler method is inadequate and the patient is unconscious. If there is marked depression of the rate and depth of respiration, a mechanical ventilator may be necessary, but before taking this step, assisted ventilation by compressing the rebreathing bag mentioned above should be tried. Oxygen concentrations of more than 30 per cent should not be given to patients with cyanosis who are suffering from carbon dioxide retention as, for example, in emphysema. The patient's respiratory centre is depressed by the high level of carbon dioxide and breathing is being stimulated solely by the hypoxia; if the hypoxia is abolished by oxygen in high concentration, the respiratory drive will be abolished and the patient will stop breathing.

Diagnosis

Once the airway has been dealt with, the doctor can obtain any history that is available. Frequently this amounts to no more than the fact that the patient collapsed in a street or in a shop. Some patients have been found collapsed in their home, where they may have been lying on the floor for prolonged periods; others may be brought in from work. Information on these patients may be obtained from the works medical or home nursing services. Information about school children can be obtained from the school or a teacher who has accompanied the child to hospital.

The simultaneous arrival of several patients who are members of a group suggests a common factor in the disorder, e.g. food poisoning or exposure to toxic fumes.

The ambulance attendants can give details of the circumstances under which the patient was found. They may bring in tablets or tablet containers found near the patient. Further information may be obtained by searching the patient's clothes. Tablets, the address of relatives, the name of the practitioner and much other information – to say nothing of the occasional bottle of spirits – may be found.

Examination follows normal clinical practice:

The patient's temperature should be taken with a low-reading thermometer to avoid missing hypothermia.

The respiratory rate may be greatly modified by various disorders. For example, it will be increased in hyperventilation tetany and may be of a Cheyne-Stokes character in cerebral haemorrhage. Barbiturate overdose with cyanosis and depression of respiration has become less frequent due to the diminished use of barbiturates by practitioners.

Irregularities in the pulse indicate fibrillation with the possibility of embolic phenomena occurring. A slow pulse will be found in heart block, cerebral haemorrhage or hypothermia. An increased pulse rate may indicate haemorrhagic or cardiovascular shock or, in the conscious patient, it may only be a manifestation of alarm at being involved in an unfamiliar situation. In this event the rate will return to normal in a short while if the patient is allowed to rest.

Significant changes in the blood pressure at the upper and lower end of the scale can provide pointers to the diagnosis, e.g. hypertension, possibly with complications or in combination with the pulse rate, suggest cardio-circulatory abnormalities.

Much can be learnt by watching the patient. Disturbances in consciousness, dyspnoea and neurological abnormalities can be assessed rapidly and easily in this manner.

The patient's ethnic origin should be noted.

Profuse sweating in a warm, flushed, confused patient suggests hypoglycaemia in contrast to the cold, clammy sweat of haemorrhagic or cardiac shock.

Thinning of the hair in elderly persons might indicate myxoedema.

Large numbers of bruises in the elderly usually suggest sub-optimal nutrition in a person living on his own. If the patient's name and address is known, information might be available from the Social Services Department.

Examination should be rapid and should cover all systems.

Inspection of the fundi should not be forgotten.

The urine should be examined, if necessary after catheterization.

Biochemical investigations may be required as a matter of urgency. Blood sugar levels can be checked rapidly with Dextrostix, while awaiting results from the laboratory. Blood gas analysis may be necessary in respiratory disorders or poisoning by salicylates. The laboratory may also be required to carry out a rapid screening of the blood when poisoning is suspected but cannot be confirmed or disproved by other methods. The blood level of the drug should also be established as soon as possible to enable definitive treatment to be commenced.

If the patient smells of alcohol, it does not necessarily mean that the patient is drunk. This is a well recognized clinical trap which most doctors fall into at one time or another. Unfortunately, laboratory examination of the blood is not such a straightforward matter as the more usual biochemical investigations but when the amount of alcohol consumed is of clinical importance, a blood sample should be taken for immediate analysis.

X-Ray examination is of limited value in the acute medical situation. Chest X-rays may reveal pathology; skull X-rays may show a shift in the position of the pineal body and, from time to time, both chest and skull X-rays may show evidence of a systemic disease, e.g. secondary carcinomatosis or myeloma.

Electro-cardiography is essential when cardiac disease is suspected. A definite abnormality is helpful, but unfortunately a normal tracing does not exclude disease. Infarction abnormalities do not develop for several hours and early confirmation of this condition may best be obtained by changes in the enzyme levels.

Treatment

Treatment should normally be limited to the minimum necessary to provide good clinical care of the patient. An Emergency Department is not the appropriate area in which to carry out detailed investigation or to initiate complex therapeutic measures. The patient will only be in the department for a short time before being admitted or discharged home and any measures used must be limited to the immediate requirements of the situation. Nevertheless, if there is proper liaison between the intaking medical firm and the Emergency Department, definite treatment can in some cases be started before the patient is sent to the ward.

Patients who are sent home should always be provided with a letter informing their practitioner about the treatment that they were given in the unit, and they should not be allowed home unless the doctor is satisfied that ill-effects will not develop either on the way or after they reach their destination.

A period of observation after treatment is a wise precaution, particularly for elderly patients, even if the only treatment required was a cup of tea.

Disposal

Correct disposal of a patient is a much more important matter than many juniors assume it to be when they start to work in an Emergency Department. The patient will be admitted to the wards in either the hospital to which he was taken or to those in a neighbouring hospital. He will be discharged to his home or that of a relative or friend, to a local authority institution or into the care of the police.

Frequently the distances involved may be considerable and transport by car, ambulance or rail may be necessary. If relatives have not accompanied the patient to hospital, they must always be advised to which hospital the patient has been admitted.

If the patient's condition is poor and transfer is unavoidable, then a nurse or doctor should accompany him, taking with them equipment that might be needed on the journey. Suitable apparatus for this purpose should always be readily available and should include intubation and oxygen equipment, a battery-operated cardioscope and defibrillator, and appropriate drugs for dealing with cardiac arrest or infusion therapy. The journey should be slow and steady. If a high speed journey with horns blaring, lights flashing and police escort is considered necessary, it is probable that the patient is unfit for the transfer. This type of journey can be guaranteed to harm the patient and may well cause a cardiac arrest in a patient suffering from a recent coronary thrombosis. If there is doubt or disagreement about the patient's fitness to be transferred, advice should be obtained from the consultant in charge.

Many patients are discharged home only after considerable thought. The chronic bed shortage may mean that some are sent home who would, under ideal conditions, be admitted. This unhappy situation places an added burden on the doctor, who must take steps to ensure that appropriate arrangements have been made for the patient's well-being after discharge. The patient who can go home and be looked after by a relative or friend is fortunate. It is only necessary to establish that the circumstances are adequate to provide the appropriate care, i.e. a frail elderly lady cannot hope to deal with a large bed-ridden elderly man. The Medical Social Worker or the Local Authority Social Worker should be asked to investigate the home situation before the patient is moved from the hospital and they may, in certain cases, be prepared to meet the patient when he arrives home.

When one member of an elderly infirm couple is taken to hospital and admission is not considered necessary, the Medical Social Worker may be able to arrange for help to be provided which will make home care of the patient a practical proposition. Such help may include relatives or neighbours. Alternatively, a home help may be provided by the local authority. The District Nurse may be asked to call and the meals on wheels service can be asked to help in providing meals of adequate quality at least once a day. In some areas the hospital authorities are introducing a twilight nursing service, which will enable nursing care to be made available for a greatly extended period during the evening and part of the night. These measures enable many patients, who would otherwise be admitted to hospital, to be cared for in the community. The general practitioner should always be advised in order that he may supervise the patient's care. If the patient does not progress satisfactorily, the practitioner may refer the patient back to the appropriate out-patient clinic or request a domiciliary visit from a consultant. The patient who lives on his own may be able to manage if similar arrangements can be made for his discharge, but it should be axiomatic that no patient should ever be allowed home unless the doctor is satisfied that all the necessary arrangements have been made for the patient's continuing care. If there is any doubt or uncertainty, the patient must be admitted until adequate arrangements are made. Sometimes patients who live on their own can be admitted to local authority hostels. These hostels only provide 'hotel facilities' and patients who are unable to dress or move about freely cannot be accommodated. Nursing care is not available and the hostels should not be asked to deal with patients who need these skills.

It is not uncommon for patients to be taken ill when they are a long way from home. This occurs frequently during the holiday season when journeys at the weekend may involve several hundred miles of motoring. When the patient is not the car driver, if admission is not necessary, he may be allowed home provided he is considered fit to stand the journey. If the patient is not fit to stand up to a long car journey, admission or a short stay in a local hotel until he has completely recovered, may be necessary. The other members of the family may require accommodation locally until the sick member has recovered. This can normally be arranged in a local hotel, many of which are used to helping the hospital with these problems. If necessary, the Medical Social Worker or the social services will be prepared to provide assistance in resolving any difficulties raised by the situation.

Similar provisions apply when the patient is unaccompanied, but the possibility of using the rail services for the journey must not be over-looked. Arrangements can easily be made with the ambulance service to take patients to, and collect them from, the railway station at each end of their journey. This is preferable to using the ambulance service for the journey, though this may be necessary if the patient has to be trans-ported on a stretcher. The modern 'open plan' design of railway carriages does not allow stretchers to be carried, except in the guard's van and, if the hospital is on part of the railway network where these carriages are in use, there may be no alternative to the use of the ambulance service. The ambulance service should only be asked to move patients outside their normal working area during normal working hours. Outside this period the service is working on an emergency only basis and long distance transfers may make the service short of staff to deal with local emergencies. Admission overnight may be required to avoid this dif-ficulty and, if problems should be encountered, the advice of the consultant should be obtained.

CARDIAC ARREST

This terminal event can develop suddenly, in a very wide variety of conditions, though it is usual to regard it as a possible complication of cases of coronary occlusion and these patients, in an Emergency Department, are always managed on an anticipatory basis to avoid delay if it should develop.

Irrespective of the cause, when it occurs the first step is to look at the clock. To be effective, treatment must be commenced within 4 minutes, though shorter periods improve the chances of re-starting the heart. If a cardiac arrest service is available in the hospital, a nurse should be asked to call for help. The doctor should confirm that arrest has occurred. Voluntary movements, including respiration, cease, cyanosis develops, arterial pulsations are absent and the heart cannot be felt or heard. The pupils, if not already dilated when the patient is first seen, will be fully dilated within a minute or two.

Treatment should commence immediately; it should not depend on the taking of an electro-cardiogram. At least two persons are required to give adequate initial treatment; one person commences external cardiac massage while the other clears the airway and ventilates the lungs.

External cardiac massage

The patient should be on a firm surface. The top of a trolley is quite adequate if the person doing the massage is able to stand on a stool or other object to gain the height necessary to perform the procedure. Placing the patient on the floor causes delay, requires extra assistance and makes the other steps more difficult to carry out.

The hand must be in the midline over the lower third of the sternum -- it should not overlap onto the abdomen or onto the costal cartilages on either side, otherwise there is a risk to the underlying viscera. If a 'karate' type of blow to the sternum does not re-start the heart, the sternum is depressed about 60 times a minute, stopping when the lungs are inflated about 10 times in the same period.

In a young person it is easy to obtain a 2.5 cm depression of the sternum, but in the elderly, because of the rigidity of the thoracic cage, the first depression frequently results in a cracking sensation due to several ribs or costal cartilages fracturing. This may create problems later, but at this stage it does assist in obtaining adequate cardiac compression, which can be confirmed by finding arterial pulsations in the neck.

Ventilation of the lungs

It cannot be emphasized too strongly that adequate ventilation of the lungs is of equally great importance as the cardiac compression. If either step is not properly executed, failure is inevitable. Experience suggests that, while cardiac compression is normally performed satisfactorily, there is still room for improvement in the use of the equipment used for pulmonary ventilation and this applies equally to medical, nursing and other staff who may be involved.

The first step is to remove any false teeth, after which the sucker is used to clear the pharynx of any foreign matter. An airway is then inserted and the head extended. Too large an airway may interfere with the fitting of a face mask. An airway which is too small may be blocked by the posterior end sitting on the back of the tongue.

In hospital practice, mouth-to-mouth breathing should not be necessary because suitable equipment to give more efficient ventilation should be available in every unit. Junior doctors must always familiarize themselves with the apparatus that is kept in the department for this purpose; this should be done in a quiet period as soon as the doctor takes up his appointment – the technique cannot be learnt in the acute situation.

The best equipment at this stage is a bag and mask. This may be of the Ambu or similar type, working independently of the oxygen supply, or an expiratory bag with face mask and valve, which requires an oxygen supply for its use. The Ambu and other types of bags which work by manual compression using atmospheric air can be given an oxygen supplement. If they are not fitted with a safety valve, the oxygen flow rate in adults should not exceed 4 litres per minute to avoid the risk of over-distension which could occur if they are held too firmly on the face.

The face mask used with the equipment should be of the correct size for the patient. A large man will require a size 5 mask, a smaller male or an adult female will usually take a size 4, with appropriate reduction in size for smaller patients. The narrow angle of the mask should fit the nose, and the cuff around the rim should be sound and not collapsed to ensure a good fit around the patient's mouth.

The thumb and index finger surround the upper surface of the mask, which is squeezed down on to the patient's face by the other fingers under the edge of the jaw. It may be necessary in edentulous patients to lift the skin of the side of the face up towards the face mask and hold it against the cuff by the ulnar border of the head. Normally it is possible to hold the mask on the patient's face with one hand while the other hand compresses the bag, though both hands may be necessary in some patients to ensure a good seal between the face and the mask.

There should not be an air leak when the lungs are inflated and the chest must be seen to expand, otherwise the procedure is not working. This is commonly due to air leaks around the mask or in the bag, or to obstruction of the pharynx caused by failure to extend the head. The airway may also be blocked by the lips or by foreign matter. If the bag has an adjustable release valve, it should be set so that it does not blow off until adequate distension of the lungs has been obtained. It may be necessary to alter the oxygen flow rate to achieve a balance between the release valve operation, filling of the bag and distension of the patient's lungs.

Adequate ventilation is easily achieved with this technique and there is no necessity to intubate. This should only be carried out when the situation is under control or prolonged mechanical ventilation is necessary.

The lungs should be inflated about 10 times a minute. Compression of the bag should be slow, steady and deliberate, avoiding rapid small compressions. The tendency to over-ventilate should be resisted, if necessary by counting or timing the rate with the help of a clock.

The next step is to set up an infusion of sodium bicarbonate. Cardiac arrest causes a metabolic acidosis, but over-infusion of the bicarbonate produces a metabolic alkalosis, which is avoided by limiting the dose to not more than 100 mM of the substance. Success is indicated by a disappearance of the cyanosis and constriction of the pupils. If these measures result in a return of the heart beat and spontaneous respiration, the cardiac massage should be discontinued and 50 per cent oxygen should be administered through a plastic face mask. If there is no response, the treatment should be discontinued after 10 minutes. If the pupils constrict and the colour improves there is no longer any urgency in the situation and it is not prejudicial to the patient to wait for experienced help to arrive in the department. The time can be occupied by setting up an electro-cardiograph or, preferably, a cardioscope, to allow continuous monitoring of the electrical activity of the heart.

Defibrillation

By definition, defibrillation can only be used if the heart is fibrillating. The coarser the degree of fibrillation, the greater the chance of success. Fine, low voltage fibrillations may be coarsened and the amplitude increased by the intracardiac injection of $0.5-1.0$ ml of $1/1000$ adrenaline.

The defibrillator is a dangerous piece of equipment, and the junior doctor should not attempt its use until he is thoroughly conversant with the operation of the particular machine in his department. In adults, an initial shock of 100 joules should be tried and, if this is unsuccessful, it should be increased to 200, and then to 400 joules. Some hospitals defibrillate patients with cardiac arrest without waiting for an ECG to be available. It is not advisable for an inexperienced doctor to use this technique; errors of diagnosis are possible and, provided the patient is being fully oxygenated and external cardiac massage is producing a good pulse, there is no urgency. An adequate cerebral circulation can be maintained for a period which is much longer than that needed to connect a cardioscope and send for the cardiac arrest team.

When using the defibrillator, it is important to ensure that nobody is touching the patient, the trolley or any equipment that may be connected to the patient. Certain cardioscopes can be left connected while the shock is administed, others need temporary disconnection; the doctor should ascertain the requirements of the apparatus that will be used in his unit.

The heart may commence beating after 1 or 2 shocks. If it does not, provided the pupils remain small, the patient's colour remains good, a pulse can be felt with each cardiac compression and the heart remains in fibrillation, defibrillation, using a 400 joules shock, should be continued. The authors have witnessed recovery in a man of 65 who was administered 26 shocks over a period of 50 minutes.

If the shock produces asystole, a sternal blow may re-start the fibrillation; alternatively, in intracardiac injection of 1.0 ml of 1/1000 adrenaline may be successful. Generally, however, recovery is very much related to the age of the patient and asystole in the acute situation has an extremely bad prognosis.

When the heart re-starts, 10 ml of a 10 per cent solution of calcium chloride should be given to strengthen the contraction. Ventilation must be continued until the patient commences to breathe spontaneously and, if the heart beats do not produce an adequate cardiac output, external cardiac massage should be continued until the heart is able to maintain the circulation without cyanosis developing.

If the patient has been given bicarbonate, the acid—base balance should be ascertained to exclude either a metabolic acidosis or a metabolic alkalosis from under- or over-infusion with sodium bicarbonate*.

There is always a risk, after successful defibrillation, of abnormal rhythms developing. Paroxysmal tachycardia or runs of ventricular extra systoles are very likely to revert to fibrillation, and a glucose drip containing 1.0 g of lignocaine per litre should be set up. The patient should be given a bolus injection of 100 mg of lignocaine intravenously and the drip adjusted to maintain a rhythm free from the abnormalities.

* A metabolic acidosis can be corrected by the administration of sodium bicarbonate, using the formula:
mM of bicarbonate required = 0.2 × body weight in kilograms
× base deficit in mM per litre.
This formula may not fully correct the deficit, but this is preferable to over-correction. After the infusion the acid-base status should be re-assessed and treated accordingly.

If the rate should indicate a complete or a partial heart block, atropine should be administered and a high oxygen concentration given through a face mask. Failure to respond indicates that pacing may be necessary.

If the treatment fails and the patient's relatives are in the department, it is the doctor's duty, accompanied by a senior nurse, to tell them of the death of the patient and to offer any help that may seem to be necessary.

CORONARY THROMBOSIS

The diagnosis in a patient who presents with the classical signs and symptoms, or the patient who has had a previous attack, will not be missed. The problem cases are those who present with ill-defined chest, arm or abdominal pains, which might be attributable to such an attack. A diagnosis may have to be reached on clinical grounds. The electrocardiogram and enzyme studies will be normal, and the patient's disposal is a source of concern.

If, on clinical grounds, there is a reasonable probability of the patient having a coronary thrombosis, admission is necessary, irrespective of the ECG findings. If the probability of a thrombosis is small, and the ECG does not show any changes, the patient should be sent home to bed and the general practioner should be advised. The practitioner will be able to arrange for any further investigations to be carried out at home if he considers it to be necessary. The relatives must be fully informed of the situation and the reasons for taking a particular course of action.

In the severe attack, the only treatment necessary in the Emergency Department is the relief of pain and the administration of oxygen. Entonox can be used as a temporary measure until morphine (10–15 mg) or another suitable narcotic, is given intravenously. Oxygen, in a 60 per cent concentration, is given by a face mask.

The patient should be transferred to the ward as soon as possible. In these patients extensive investigation is contra-indicated in an Emergency Department and the sooner the patient is in bed the better the chances of his recovery.

ACUTE LEFT VENTRICULAR FAILURE

These patients present in a highly distressed condition. They are dyspnoeic to a degree which prevents any history being obtained; they sit up and lean forwards and are sweating profusely from the muscular effort involved. They are dusky grey in colour with cyanosed lips, ears and mucous membranes; froth, due to pulmonary oedema, may be present.

Morphine (10–15 mg) may, by relieving the apprehension, produce a marked improvement in the patient's condition.

If there appears to be an element of bronchial spasm present, 0.25 g of Aminophylline, should be given intravenously. Administration must be slow because cardiac arrest may develop if it is given too rapidly.

Oxygen (30 per cent) will be of help and, if the dyspnoea is severe, the concentration should be increased to 60 per cent.

Diuretics, e.g. Frusemide, are also of value in the acute attack if pulmonary oedema is present.

DIABETES

Routine urine testing is essential in all cases of collapse. The classical diabetic coma with ketosis is a rare event in the Emergency Department, but most departments will diagnose one or two cases of diabetes every year in patients who were unaware that they had this disorder. Admission of these patients is essential.

More frequently patients are admitted with acute hypoglycaemia. They are usually unconscious, but fortunately the information that they are being treated with insulin or oral therapy usually comes in with the patient via a relative, friend or workmate. Hypoglycaemia should always be considered in apparently fit persons who suddenly lose consciousness. This conclusion will be reinforced if there is a history of confusion or irrational behaviour, needing restraint, in a previously normal individual. The patient may, if there is marked restlessness needing restraint, be sweating profusely.

The urine should be examined after catheterization. The patient's possessions may reveal evidence of diabetic therapy and Dextrostix examination may suggest hypoglycaemia. Blood should be sent to the laboratory for glucose estimation, but the therapeutic test of 25–50 g of dextrose given intravenously should not be delayed. Prolonged hypoglycaemia causes cerebral damage, which can result in the death of the patient.

Glucagon should not be used unless glucose therapy cannot be given; it depends for its action on mobilizing liver glycogen and if this is low, there will be little or no response and recovery will be delayed.

If intravenous glucose is not available, 20 g of glucose can be given through a stomach tube in a 5 per cent concentration. No attempt should be made to administer the glucose orally unless the patient is able to swallow.

Recovery should be followed by a carbohydrate meal and the reason for the attack should be investigated.

Patients on long-acting insulins raise difficulties and may require referral to the Diabetic Unit if they appear to be getting out of control.

The patient should never be discharged without a period of observation and a blood glucose estimation should be carried out unless the doctor can be sure that the condition will not recur. This decision is based on the nature and dosage of the insulin, the time of the attack, the reliability of the diabetic history and the commonsense (and availability) of the persons who will be associating with the patient after discharge.

From time to time patients attempt suicide using massive doses of insulin. Initial recovery occurs rapidly with glucose, but as they are unlikely to be truthful and may well have injected themselves with a great deal more long-acting insulin than they will admit to, there is every possibility that the hypoglycaemia will recur. Constant monitoring of the blood glucose level and a glucose drip, if appropriate, is the only safe method to deal with these patients.

POISONING

In adults the majority of cases of poisoning are the result of attempted suicide. In contrast to children, relatively few cases are accidental and, of these, many follow industrial accidents and involve uncommon substances whose precise effects may be difficult to ascertain.

In the past decade there has been a change in the pattern of self-poisoning. The changeover to North Sea gas has resulted in a fall of the death rate from gas poisoning. Similarly, barbiturate overdose has dropped significantly and its place has been taken by the new psychotropic drugs. Unfortunately, the treatment of an overdose of the more modern drugs is less satisfactory due to their more complex mode of action. The drug manufacturers must also take some of the blame for the present situation. One widely distributed pain relieving drug has been found to be addictive to certain patients. Another, composed of a common analgesic in combination with a different drug of doubtful value offers little benefit over the basic substance. Indeed, the only result of this approach of polypharmacy is to increase the dangers of an overdose by adding to the basic drug risk of liver failure, a second and immediate danger of cardiac arrest, which can occur before or soon after the patient reaches hospital.

The junior doctor should be conscious of his responsibilities in relation to the use and abuse of drugs and should not allow himself to be talked into using new and untried drugs by the blandishments of the drug companies' representatives. It is a safe precept to assume that every drug powerful enough to produce an effect on a patient will, on occasions, produce totally unexpected adverse effects. When one is dealing with patients whose medical record and personality are unknown, it is always safest to rely on well known drugs whose beneficial effects have stood the test of time.

The number of substances now available is so large that it is essential that suitable reference books are available in each department. A list of suitable volumes is given in Appendix 4, but help in both the identification and treatment of the substance can be obtained from the hospital pharmacists. The fire service holds literature about substances that might be carried by road. Agricultural colleges may be of assistance when plant life is involved. The Ministry of Agriculture or the Factory Inspectorate can also be of help, but the most useful advice in a medical context can be obtained from the Poisons Information Centres, whose details are listed in the Appendix. These centres are able to assist in the identification and advise in the management of poisoning from drugs, chemicals and other substances.

Unless the clinical situation is acute the junior doctor should always endeavour to find out as much as possible from the reference books in the department before contacting the Poisons Centre. Familiarity with the reference literature is important, because many cases are not clear-cut and final decisions may have to be based on a clinical assessment, for which the fullest information, including the alternatives, must be immediately available to the medical staff.

Management

The management of a case of suspected poisoning in the Emergency Department falls into stages.

Stage I – Immediate resuscitation

This stage is not necessary in the majority of cases, but from time to time immediate action is necessary, irrespective of the presumed nature of the poisoning.

If the patient's breathing is depressed, oxygen should be administered through a face mask.

If the patient is not breathing, artificial ventilation, using an Ambu bag or a bag and face mask with oxygen, or intubation and mechanical ventilation – in this order – should be commenced.

Tracheal toilet, using a sucker, should be carried out.

If circulatory collapse is present, plasma expanders should be used.

The seriously ill patient should always be connected to a cardioscope.

A blood sample should be taken for laboratory screening and estimation, and an arterial blood sample should be obtained if the patient's metabolic state is thought to require investigation.

If the substance has contaminated the skin and clothing, after removal of the clothing the skin should be irrigated profusely with large volumes of water or an appropriate neutralizing agent (*see* Appendix 2).

Once the acute situation is over, Stage II follows.

Stage II – Identification

In most patients the necessity for Stage I management does not arise, and the doctor can start immediately with the identification of the poison. The pharmacy is of great assistance in the identification of tablets which are otherwise loose or in inappropriate containers. It is, however, more usual for the tablet container to be brought into the hospital with the patient. Sometimes a large collection of tablets is brought in, and deciding which drug has been consumed is a matter of guesswork rather than logic (*Figure 23.1*).

If the container is available, the name of the drug should be written on the label. If not, information may be available from the chemist who supplied the prescription. Alternatively, the general practitioner may be able to assist. The formulation of proprietary products can be found in *Martindale*, and the essential ingredient in agricultural and gardening products can usually be identified by reference to the publication *Approved Products for Farmers and Growers* (*see* Appendix 4).

Industrial substances require a reference to be made to appropriate books and possibly to the Poisons Centre, who possess considerable

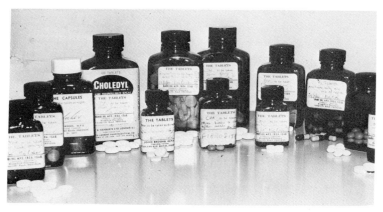

Figure 23.1. A collection of tablets brought in with a patient who had taken an overdose. Identification of the drug consumed was not possible

information (made available in confidence by the manufacturers) about various products which are used both in the home and in industry.

If poisoning is suspected but there is no external evidence of any drug consumption, the laboratory should be asked to carry out a screening for the common groups of drugs. Aspirin, paracetamol, barbiturates and various neuroleptic drugs can be identified quickly and quantitative estimations can be made if this is relevant.

Alcohol is a common extra finding in drug overdose; the use of apparatus giving direct blood levels is very helpful in this respect.

In most cases it is usually possible, though it may take a considerable time, to establish the drug or probable substance that has been taken. If this is not possible, treatment must be symptomatic.

Stage III – Primary elimination

In this stage the primary removal of the poison is undertaken. This may be coupled with steps to neutralize the drug. Skin contaminants have already been removed as part of the initial reception procedures, and injected poisons cannot be removed in the Emergency Department. The only decision to be made is the necessity or otherwise for a stomach wash-out to be undertaken. A stomach wash-out should not be carried out for poisoning by any petroleum product or corrosive chemical, nor should it be undertaken in an unconscious patient unless the airway has been protected by a cuffed endotracheal tube. There is little point in attempting to remove drugs by this procedure after 4 hours from the time of consumption, except for aspirin and tricyclic antidepressants. These drugs are exceptional because significant amounts of the drug can be removed for several hours longer than this period.

The largest possible stomach tube should be used. A soft rubber 30 gauge English (Jacques) tube is suitable. The large size enables the stomach contents to be removed without the tube becoming blocked and also makes it difficult to enter the trachea in error. The tube should be passed with the patient lying on one side with the table tilted into the head-down position. A sucker, which should be tested before commencing the procedure, must be available.

If estimations of the drugs in the stomach are required, the first specimen obtained through the tube should be used for this purpose.

Large quantities of fluid should be used and the operation continued until it is returned clear.

In most cases there is little point in leaving any so-called antidotes in the stomach prior to removal of the tube. The number of substances recommended for this purpose is as high as the number of solutions recommended for use during wash-out, and there is little evidence that it benefits the patient. There are, however, certain drugs, of which desferrioxamine is an example, which must be left in the stomach after removal of the tube. The reference material will indicate the circumstances when this practice is necessary and will also indicate if there are any specific antidotes or chemical agents which can reasonably be expected to benefit the patient.

The junior doctor should realize that there are very few substances which can be expected to produce a significant change in the patient's condition while in the Emergency Department. Most of the patients who develop toxic effects do so after they have left the Emergency Department, thus becoming the responsibility of the Medical Unit.

Stage IV – Disposal

It is usually accepted that patients who have been treated for self-poisoning should always be admitted. This is to ensure that they do not develop toxic effects or make a further attempt at suicide. It is also recommended that all cases of suicide should be seen by a psychiatrist. This is normally arranged by the in-patient firm under whose care the patient is admitted. This approach may on occasions be modified if the patient has only taken an insignificant amount of the drug. If the patient can be discharged into the care of a responsible relative, who is able to provide adequate supervision, it may be thought safe to allow the patient home, provided the psychiatric service is informed before the patient's discharge from hospital and the general practitioner is notified.

If the psychiatric services have a constant presence in the hospital, they may well be prepared to see the patient immediately after the initial treatment has been concluded when in-patient medical supervision is not required. This ideal arrangement is, unfortunately, less frequent than the normal case, where the psychiatric services are based in another hospital. As a result, communication problems do arise and, when there is concern about the patient's mental well-being in relation to his treatment in the Accident and Emergency Department, the only safe approach is to consult the duty psychiatrist directly.

The 'chronic' or recurrent case of self-poisoning, who appears regularly in the department after the consumption of varying amounts of a different drug on each occasion, is primarily a psychiatric problem. The management in the Accident Department must be carried out as if the patient were making his first visit. Subsequently, it is a problem for the psychiatric services, who should be consulted about the difficulties and problems that the situation is causing for both the doctor and the patient.

HYPOTHERMIA

This condition normally occurs in young babies and the elderly. Nevertheless, it can arise in young fit adults during their everyday activities. For example, it has been seen in a young man, with inadequate clothing, riding his motorcycle on a day when the temperature dropped suddenly to below zero. It has also been seen in a telephone linesman who was working in windy, sub-zero conditions on top of a telephone pole.

The routine use of low-reading thermometers is essential if cases are not to be missed and the junior doctor should always exercise care in the diagnosis of death during inclement weather. Patients who take an overdose of barbitruates and subsequently expose themselves to the weather may, if it is cold, develop profound hypothermia, which has all the clinical appearances of death.

Death should only be confirmed after electro-cardiograph examination in patients who are suffering from exposure or who may have been exposed to low temperatures in unheated houses. Slow re-warming by preventing heat loss is essential for elderly patients, whose heart should be monitored during the process.

Fit, young adults suffering from acute hypothermia may be treated by rapid re-warming. This is not free from danger because the application of warmth may dilate the skin capillaries while the body core temperature remains low. If the blood pressure falls, intravenous fluid may be necessary to restore the circulating blood volume to an adequate level. Because of this, slow re-warming using special heat-retaining blankets, or normal blankets in a warm room, is preferable to attempting to raise the temperature rapidly by the use of external sources of heat.

TROPICAL DISEASES

The possibility of meeting this group of diseases is significantly higher than a decade ago, due to the speeding up of travel caused by air transport and the increase in the immigrant population, many of whom are from areas where these diseases are prevalent. Before air travel reached its present level, most diseases developed before the patient, travelling by sea, reached this country, but now symptoms may not arise for several days after the patient's arrival and, because of unfamiliarity, delays in diagnosis are common.

About 1500 cases of malaria were reported in the UK in 1977, and in one department during that year a case of leprosy and an infection from a Tombu fly were seen. This latter condition is caused by the insect laying an egg under the skin; this develops into a maggot, which causes a boil-like swelling. The maggot, similar to that of a bluebottle fly, can be removed from the centre of the 'boil'.

Most UK doctors are inexperienced in the diagnosis and management of tropical diseases, though many immigrant doctos have extensive experience of these disorders and the need for their assistance should always be considered if there is a possibility of such a disorder being present.

The suspicion of a tropical disease is raised when a patient is taken ill shortly after returning from an area where such diseases are endemic. The initial symptoms are not clearly defined, tending to suggest a 'flu' like illness. A high fever with rigors suggests malaria and a thick blood film should always be taken, as this may give immediate information about the diagnosis. If other diseases are suspected, the assistance of the laboratory services should be obtained because special investigations may be necessary. Patients who suffer from recurrent malaria may provide the doctor with the diagnosis, but if there is uncertainty little harm will be caused by treating the patient for malaria. Other diseases require time for the completion of laboratory tests and malaria, the commonest disorder, will respond rapidly to treatment whereas, if another disease is present, the patient's condition will not be prejudiced in any way.

Patients in whom a tropical disease is suspected should normally be admitted. Advice can always be obtained from the hospitals for tropical diseases in London and Liverpool and in some cases it may be advisable for the patient to be transferred to one of these centres. This decision, however, should not be taken by the junior doctor, who should always seek his consultant's advice before contacting these centres.

IATROGENIC DISEASE

This is a disease caused by doctors while treating (*Figure 23.2*) or investigating (*Figures 23.3* and *23.4*) patients.

Since 1948, there has been a passive increase in the range of drugs available to treat patients. Surgical techniques have changed, new techniques have been introduced, and methods of investigation have become increasingly complex and invasive. The demand for medical care has increased and consequently more people than ever before are exposed to the risks that inevitably follow evolutionary changes of this nature.

The classical example in recent times of unanticipated complications following the use of a new drug is the thalidomide tragedy. Fortunately, major incidents of this nature are uncommon and much effort has been devoted to minimizing the risk of such effects occurring in the future. Nevertheless, the junior doctor would do well to remember that, despite the care devoted to ensuring the safety of drugs, it is inevitable that patients will from time to time react in an unexpected manner.

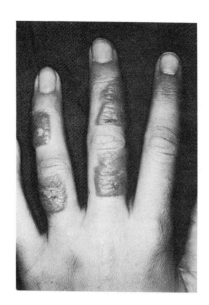

Figure 23.2. Dermatitis caused by sensitivity to strapping used during treatment of a fractured finger

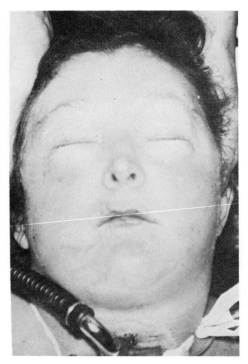

Figure 23.3. Gross facial oedema caused by surgical emphysema following bronchography performed by cricothyroid puncture. The patient also exhibited iodine sensitivity to the contrast medium. During tracheostomy, a small flap valve, caused by the needle in the cricothyroid, was revealed by air bubbles appearing at each expiration. Bronchial lavage to remove part of the contrast medium was possible through the tracheostomy

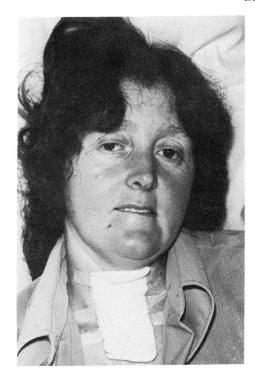

Figure 23.4. The same patient (as shown in Figure 23.3*) 4 days after the facial swelling had subsided*

In an Accident Department certain hazards, for example sensitivity to antibiotics and the reactions following the use of antitetanus serum prepared from horses, are well recognized. A less well recognized therapeutic complication is a sensitivity developing to chloromycetin eye ointment. Panophthalmitis, requiring removal of the eye, may follow the careless use of steroids in certain inflammatory eye conditions.

Subcutaneous atrophy may follow the prolonged use of topical steroids and, if this atrophy affects the face, it can be, to both patient and doctor, a permanent reminder of the hazards of modern therapy.

In an Accident Department there are frequent changes of medical and nursing staff. The patients are not known to the doctors, who frequently have to work under very great pressure. It is therefore essential that preference should always be given to methods of treatment which have a high safety factor and drugs should only be used when there is clear indication for their use. New drugs and techniques should be introduced with care, keeping a careful watch on the patient, and not until the doctor is satisfied with their safety and effectiveness should they be introduced into regular clinical use.

24

The Accident Officer and the Law

The junior doctor starting to work in an Accident and Emergency Department is always worried about the legal problems that working in such a unit can produce. Apart from his own position and the difficulties in which he may find himself as a result of his own errors of omission or commission, the complexities of the law in relation to his patients are always a source of anxiety. He feels vulnerable in respect of complaints which may be made, sometimes without good grounds, and unless help from more experienced doctors is readily available, he tends to practise defensive medicine by X-raying patients unnecessarily or bringing them back for review at unnecessarily short intervals.

NEGLIGENCE

The possibility of being sued for negligence is very much in the forefront of the junior's concern, yet it is a situation which applies to all doctors during their clinical work and, even in the casualty situation, should not be allowed to influence the treatment of a patient. Negligence can be defined as: 'a failure to use reasonable skill and care, when treating a patient, which results in damage to that patient'. Once a doctor starts to treat a patient, he undertakes to use reasonable skill and care. The law recognizes that no doctor can have a high degree of skill in every specialty, and therefore the standard of care depends on the experience and position held by the doctor. From this it follows that the junior doctor in an Emergency Department will not be expected to possess the knowledge and experience of the consultant in charge of the department. As a hypothetical example, a junior doctor missing a dislocated semilunar bone would not be held to exhibit the degree of negligence that the consultant would display if he missed the same injury.

The defence against negligence is not very simple, but basically requires that the doctor should take a good history, make an adequate examination and **record** his findings and treatment in sufficient detail to enable the situation to be reconstructed at a later date. (These notes should also be decipherable without calling in a handwriting expert.)

264

Reference has previously been made in earlier chapters to the importance of adequate documentation. The annual reports of the defence societies highlight the problems that are raised by a failure in documentation and, if a doctor is sued for negligence, a defence is only possible if the notes, made at the time or very shortly thereafter, can be produced to support the treatment or advice given to the patient. When the mechanics of the injury, given in the history, and the examination do not suggest that a fracture is present, provided the reasons for not X-raying the patient are clearly set out, a good defence against negligence is possible. In contrast, a single-line comment on the records, without an adequate (and relevant) history or examination, made in an illegible and unsigned scrawl, cannot be regarded as an adequate assessment of the patient and would be of little help in defending an accusation of negligence.

It must be realized that many complaints and legal interventions are made a considerable time after the patient attended hospital. In a department which sees many thousands of patients every year, the written record is the only adequate means of protecting both the doctor and the patient. Memory under these circumstances is totally unreliable.

It is also good practice to record any untoward or unusual incident that happens to a patient. Legal action against doctors is comparatively rare, but complaints, particularly in the present climate, can be a source of considerably worry and it is always best to record full details of incidents while they are fresh in one's memory.

The defence societies, whose membership is compulsory for all National Health Service medical and dental staff, should always be contacted either by telephone or in writing immediately a doctor becomes aware that he is likely to be involved in a complaint or legal action about his treatment of a patient. They will advise the doctor about ethical matters, the handling of complaints against him, problems arising with the administration and the conditions under which he has to work. When major problems do arise, the junior should seek the help of his consultant who will, if necessary, work closely with the defence society on his junior's behalf.

COMPLAINTS

Many complaints, as opposed to legal actions, arise from a failure of the doctor to communicate adequately with the patient. The atmosphere of a busy Accident and Emergency Department is frightening, even to intelligent and responsible persons. Many patients attending Accident and Emergency Departments are of restricted ability and intelligence or are overwhelmed by the circumstances in which they find themselves.

The doctor must realize that patients do not react normally under these conditions and he should always deal sympathetically with them and satisfy himself that they appreciate what has happened, what treatment they are to have and what arrangements have been made for follow-up. These details should always be entered into the notes in case enquiries are made in the future.

VIOLENCE

The aggressive patient does raise difficulties. The doctor should restrain his natural tendencies to reply in kind. Aggression begets aggression and if a sympathetic approach, possibly helped by a member of the nursing staff, is adopted, most patients will quieten down and allow themselves to be treated in the normal way. However, if a patient becomes violent, abusive or aggressive, causes a hazard to other patients or the staff and refuses to leave the department, the police should be asked to remove the offender.

Care must be taken to establish, as far as possible, that such a patient is not suffering from a medical or surgical condition, e.g. hypoglycaemia or a head injury which requires treatment; this group of patients are not responsible for their actions and should be treated appropriately. The uncontrollable drunk, however, may create a dangerous situation for other patients and, if he is not amenable to reason, it is preferable that he should be removed by the police if he will not remove himself. Treatment can always be given when he has sobered up.

Violent patients except, for example, hypoglycaemic cases, should never be given any drugs to control their violence. To do so without their permission will constitute an assault. Of more significance, however, is the danger of giving a patient a powerful drug without any knowledge of any other drugs they may have consumed. The doctor should always be aware that physical restraint of a patient is illegal and whenever this is necessary he should be fully prepared to justify this action.

REFUSAL OF TREATMENT

If a patient refuses to accept treatment or admission to hospital, he must be allowed to discharge himself, preferably after signing an appropriate form accepting the responsibility for his action. If he will not sign such a form, this should be indicated on the case sheet, which must be counter-signed by a witness, who may be either another doctor or a senior nurse. When a person under 16 refuses to accept treatment, the parents should be contacted and asked to attend the department.

When parents refuse to allow essential treatment, e.g. blood transfusion or an operation, to be carried out on a child, possibly for religious reasons, the consultant in charge should be contacted as it may be necessary to take the child into the care of the local authority.

CONSENT FOR OPERATION

A standard form is in use in most hospitals for this purpose. It is important that the reason for any surgical procedure should be explained to the patient by the doctor. The doctor advises the patient and it is the patient's privilege to accept or reject this advice. Whenever possible, some idea of the future course of the condition should be given to the patient before the procedure is carried out. The patient knows what to expect and, if a perfect result is unlikely, the patient will accept this more easily if he is aware of the position from the beginning.

Persons over the age of 16 can sign their own consent form but, whenever possible in young persons, every effort should be made to contact the parents before the operation. If the patient does not wish this to be done, the decision should be accepted if the patient is over 16. Under the age of 16, the person in charge of the child, e.g. a school teacher or a scout master if the child is away at camp, can sign the consent for operation if it is not practical to contact the patents in time.

In cases of extreme urgency, e.g. an extra-dural haemorrhage, the doctor must be prepared to carry out the necessary treatment even without permission being obtained. This situation is fortunately not common, but it can occur, particularly after road traffic accidents and, if delay in obtaining parental consent would jeopardize the well-being of the patient, the doctor would be failing in his duty to the patient by accepting such a delay in carrying out the treatment. Equally, there is no urgency when treating closed fractures without circulatory or neurological complications and such patients can be given holding treatment, e.g. splints and sedation until proper consent is obtained.

CONFIDENTIALITY

The medical profession is privileged by being given information from patients that they would not make available to any other person. In return, patients are entitled to have this confidential information about themselves held under secure conditions and not made available to third persons without their consent. The rule of secrecy may have to be broken when statutory requirements, such as the notification of infectious diseases or the certification of death, have to be completed.

With the patient's permission, information may be disclosed to any third party, such as an employer. When a solicitor acting on behalf of the patient requests information, permission is implied, but a report should never be given to a solicitor or insurance company who does not act for the patient without written permission being obtained. In a Court of Law confidential information about the patient may have to be given if the judge directs that the doctor disclose such information. As a result of the McIver decision made in May 1978 in the House of Lords, if a plaintiff or his solicitor supplies appropriate reasons to a court, they can obtain an order for the disclosure of the hospital records directly to the solicitor. This decision is of importance to the doctor working in an Emergency Department. It emphasizes the necessity to keep good, accurate, legible records and indirectly highlights the need to avoid writing any derogatory comments on the notes which might reflect adversely on his colleagues or on the patient.

If any comments are considered necessary, they should always take the form of factual observations. The use of two- or three-word opinions should be avoided because the doctor would be unlikely to remember the grounds on which he based his opinion by the time the case reached court, and there is also a possibility that a conclusion – as opposed to an observation – might turn out to be wrong. A situation of this nature would reflect little credit on the doctor and could well prejudice the outcome of any proceedings in which he had been asked by the plaintiff or the defendant to give medical evidence.

The rule of confidentiality also extends to specimens taken from the patient. For example, vomit must not be given to the police for forensic examination without the patient's consent, nor must blood samples be taken for the police without consent being given. In general, the safest approach to the problem of confidentiality is not to give out any information about the patient without his or her permission. This generalization holds good for the majority of circumstances and, when in doubt, the doctor should ask his consultant.

There are 2 areas where problems can arise, usually unexpectedly, and rapid decisions may have to be made:

1. The press ring up to enquire about patients who have been injured after accidents. If the injuries are the result of a road traffic accident, it is wisest to refer the enquirer to the police to obtain the information. If the injuries have followed industrial or other accidents, the hospital administration, during the day-time, should be asked to deal with the enquiry. At nights, or when the administration is not available, provided the relatives have been notified a generalized statement as to the patient's condition and injuries can be given. Specific details of the injuries should be avoided and

the doctor should not be persuaded by a highly skilled enquirer to enlarge upon the minimal details.

If several victims have been admitted following an incident which appears to be newsworthy, there will be considerable press activity and the hospital administration must be prepared to establish an enquiry bureau, irrespective of the day or time.

2. Police enquiries after road traffic accidents are necessary, *inter alia*, for statistical purposes and there is no harm in giving appropriate details. If the patient's condition is serious, apart from being prepared to assist in notifying relatives, it may be necessary for further enquiries to be made into the cause of the accident.

When a patient has been seriously assaulted, it may be necessary, provided the time can be spared from the clinical situation, to discuss the injuries with the senior officer in charge of the case. Rapid action by the police may result in the speedy arrest of the assailant and, when the patient's injuries are serious or liable to result in death or serious incapacity, the community has a right to expect that all possible steps will be taken to capture the person responsible. If the patient's condition allows, it may be necessary to allow the police to have a short interview with the patient; they are always co-operative in these cases and will limit their interview to the length of time allowed by the doctor.

If the injured patient is the assailant or is likely to be charged with a serious offence, the police will insist on one of their officers remaining with the patient at all times. This requirement must be accepted by the staff; it can, if the patient is violent, be of considerable assistance to them in controlling the situation with minimal risk to other patients, staff and equipment.

DRUG ADDICTS

Patients suffering from an overdose of any drug of addiction are ill and should be treated appropriately, if necessary by admission.

The registered drug addict who obtains his opiate drugs from a special clinic and comes to the department with withdrawal symptoms, or claiming he has lost or broken his ampoule of morphia or heroin, should be handled sympathetically but carefully. There is a ready market for these drugs and, whenever possible, the Drug Addiction Clinic should be contacted. In many cases it will be found that the alleged story does not stand up and the advice of the clinic should be acted upon.

If the patient is suffering from acute withdrawal symptoms, an injection of methadone may be given and the patient advised to report back to the next available clinic. If such patients keep coming back with differing stories as to how they lost their drugs, or if the number of addicts begins to show a progressive increase, the doctor must consider whether or not he is handling the situation in the correct manner and advice should be obtained from his consultant.

When a young person under 16 is brought into hospital under the influence of drugs, the necessary treatment should be given. The relatives or guardian should be interviewed. If the drugs were obtained from home, appropriate advice should be given about the care of the drugs and the assistance of the general practitioner and, possibly, a psychiatrist sought for the further management of the problem. If the drugs were obtained illegally, the parents should be advised to discuss the matter with the police drug squad, who are very anxious to trace drug pushers and are quite prepared to discuss the problem with the parents without taking any action against the patient.

Pethidine addicts are not infrequent. They may present as cases of renal colic and, on examination, the abdomen often shows external evidence of previous surgery. Usually they arrive late at night and frequently have no local address. It is important not to miss a genuine case and the best approach is to handle them in a fully professional manner. A detailed past history should be obtained, including the names of the last hospitals to which the patient was admitted and the names and adresses of any practitioners the patient has recently consulted. An attempt should be made to contact the hospitals and practitioners by telephone. The information received by such enquiries invariably reveals the genuine case, which contrasts markedly with the lack of information available about the addict. In the latter case the practitioners' names are usually fictitious and there is no record of the patient having been admitted to any of the institutions which he names. When these facts are pointed out to the patient, there is an extremely rapid resolution of the complaints, followed by an equally rapid, voluntary removal of the patient from the department.

PSYCHIATRIC PROBLEMS

Patients with acute psychiatric disorders are often extremely difficult to manage.

The acute hysterical paralysis, while relatively uncommon, is a psychiatric emergency and arrangements should be made for the patient to be seen urgently in a Psychiatric Clinic.

The patient who is determined to commit suicide must never be discharged home. Medical or surgical conditions will require appropriate treatment, if necessary as an in-patient, but those in whom admission is not required should be referred to the psychiatrist immediately. The telephone is the appopriate method of consultation in these circumstances and the psychiatrist's advice should be followed. When patients are suffering from psychiatric disorders for which the doctor considers that admission to a mental hospital would be appropriate, it is best to consult with the duty psychiatrist. The routine for dealing with such patients varies widely throughout the country, and the local routines are always the most expeditious in resolving the problems.

From time to time the advice received may not appear appropriate for the patient's needs. Psychiatrists are reluctant to admit or treat patients whom they do not consider will benefit from their care and, if the advice is that the patient should be discharged, the junior doctor must accept this advice, provided it comes from a senior member of the psychiatric services. He should not, however, forget to discuss the matter with his own consultant if he is still uneasy about the implications of any advice which he may have received.

Certification of the patient requires the presence of a Social Worker and 1 or 2 doctors, one of whom must be approved under the Mental Health Act for the purpose, depending on which section of the Act is being used for the purpose.

LEGAL PROCEDURES

The coroner

The coroner occupies a unique place in the legal structure of the country. The post dates back many centuries and, within his own court, he has considerable power and the ability to lay down certain procedures which may supplement the statutory requirements of his office.

Apart from occasional forays into such esoteric subjects as buried treasure, his primary function is to inquire into cases of sudden or unexpected death and establish how and by what means the deceased met his death.

In recent years, fortunately perhaps for the medical profession, coroners have become less liable to use their office to express their personal views about situations in which they feel a strong interest. In times past, such an approach by a self-opinionated coroner could have a very serious effect on medical morale, because staff found that they were being publicly subjected to ill-informed criticism, which they were unable to counter because of the unique power of the office. Nowadays, the comments tend to be much more informed, more balanced, and usually very relevant to the situation.

Recommendations from a Coroner's Court carry considerable weight and, in the hospital context, can produce speedy action to prevent the recurrence of a situation which would necessitate the holding of an inquest.

The law requires that death occurring under certain circumstances, or from specific diseases, should be reported to the coroner. To report a death to the coroner, the details of the death are notified by telephone to the coroner's officer, who is usually a Police Officer attached to the coroner for this purpose. If he should not be available, the death can be reported to the local police station. In certain hospitals, a member of the administrative staff is responsible for such notifications, and it is always wise for the junior doctor to ascertain the local routine for dealing with such matters.

The following deaths should be notified to the coroner. All cases where death is the result of violence, unnatural causes or is due to natural causes but the doctor cannot certify death because he has not previously treated the patient. Deaths occurring during anaesthesia, as a result of surgery or attributable to the treatment should also be notified. The coroner should also be notified of all deaths occurring in mental hospitals, prisons, in persons suffering from prescribed occupational diseases, certain toxic industrial substances and when the person is in receipt of a war pension or pension for an industrial disease.

When the patient dies in the Accident Department, it is the doctor's responsibility to ensure that the coroner is notified. When the doctor merely confirms death and the body is removed to the mortuary, the responsibility for the notification belongs to the authorities responsible for the mortuary services. However, when death appears to be due to violence inflicted upon the deceased by another person, it is advisable that the police should be notified immediately and instructions given that the body and clothing should not be disturbed in any way, other than to establish that death has occurred.

From time to time the junior doctor will be unsure as to the appropriate action he should take in relation to a death. Staff in A & E Departments should never be required to give a death certificate, though such certificates can be given by the general practitioner who has been looking after the patient. When there is uncertainty, the junior doctor should seek the help of his consultant or ring up the coroner personally and ask for advice. Usually the coroner's officer or clerk will be able to assist and, if not, they will contact the coroner and ask for his instructions.

If the doctor feels that his conduct is in any way likely to be criticized at an inquest, he should contact his defence society immediately. He should also write out a full report on the incident which is causing him concern. Memory is fallible and the only safe approach is to set out the facts on paper as soon as possible after the incident.

Courts

Attendance at court is always a worrying affair for the junior doctor. Anyone working in an A & E Department comes into frequent contact with the results of personal violence. In these cases he is required to attend and give evidence as a witness of fact. That is to say, his evidence relates to matters which he observed in the course of examination and treatment of the patient. He will be required to attend the Magistrates' Court, which is the lowest tier of court in the structure.

Preparation for giving his evidence starts with a Police Officer taking a statement. This is a formal document, usually written in longhand, setting out the doctor's name, qualifications and post. It then deals with the facts of the case as known to the doctor and terminates with a conclusion, which may indicate his opinion as to the degree of violence used, the severity of the injury, the possibility of permanent incapacity and an indication that the injuries are compatible with the use of a certain implement or weapon. The statement is then signed by the doctor.

He will then be notified by the police of the time and date of the hearing. On arrival at court he should report to the usher, if he is not recognized by the constable involved, who will advise him where he can wait until his case is due to he heard. When he is required to give evidence, he enters the witness box and takes the oath to speak the truth in a manner appropriate to his religious belief.

He will then be taken through his statement by the prosecutor, who may be either a Police Officer or a solicitor. He will then be asked questions by the defence solicitor. It is important that his evidence is given clearly, and it should be addressed to the Magistrates. The doctor should never hesitate, if skilled questioning draws a false conclusion, to indicate that, in his view, the conclusion is erroneous. It is equally important to confine his comments to matters about which he is confident. Solicitors are skilled in the art of cross-examination and the inexperienced doctor can find himself in a situation where he is admitting that what he has just said in evidence is not really as accurate as he had imagined before he made his comments.

If the crime is of greater magnitude than can be dealt with by Magistrates, it will be heard in the Crown Court. This is a court presided over by a judge with a jury, where the examination and cross-examination is carried out by barristers. The doctor's statement will be taken on a special form; it may be typed out on the form and he will have to sign each page. The evidence is initially heard by Magistrates at committal proceedings, where the decision is made that the evidence justifies the accused being sent to the Crown Court for trial. The doctor is not usually required to attend these proceedings.

He will later be given a subpoena, that is a legal document requiring him to attend the court and give evidence in the case of Regina v. the accused. It is not advisable to ignore such a document, but the courts are always sympathetic if there are times when a doctor could not attend, provided that the problem has been discussed in good time. The police are the appropriate persons to contact if there are any difficulties, such as examinations, likely to arise at about the time of the hearing.

The procedure in court follows a similar, though a slightly more formal, course to that in the Magistrates' Court. The evidence should be given clearly and directed towards the judge and jury. Barristers are even more skilled than solicitors in putting words in the mouths of inexperienced doctors and the only sound advice is to answer the questions simply and never volunteer any information. This latter step has been the downfall of many doctors in the witness box, irrespective of their experience, age and professional standing.

Despite the rather worrying surroundings, the whole procedure is conducted quietly and with great politeness. The judge is, in some ways, in the position of a referee and, if the questioning appears to be getting unreasonable, or if the conclusions drawn by the barrister are inaccurate, the fact should be made known to the judge.

Judges are addressed as 'My Lord' or 'Your Honour'. The former applies to a High Court Judge who is on circuit, i.e. taking the serious cases in the courts around the circuit. The latter applies to a less senior judge, who spends his time entirely in a restricted number of courts, hearing all but the most serious cases. Occasionally a recorder, who is a barrister 'acting up' as a judge may take the case. The precise mode of address can be ascertained by listening to the barristers when they address the judge. Magistrates are addressed as 'Sir' or 'Madam'.

Even in Crown Court proceedings, the junior doctor will be acting as a witness to fact. An expert witness is usually a senior member of the profession with special skills in a certain field who has been asked to study and comment about the medical evidence. Such a witness may be used by both the prosecution and defence, and the junior should feel relieved that the barristers reserve their main attacks for these persons.

The drunken driver

It is an offence to drive with a blood alcohol level above 80 mg per 100 ml of blood. Parliament recognized the difficultues that the introduction of the breathalyser and blood and urine testing would produce for Accident and Emergency Departments and special provisions were introduced to avoid the public thinking that hospital staff were involved with the police in detecting and subsequently appearing for the prosecution in cases of driving under the influence of drink. It is important that the medical staff are aware of the requirements of the Road Traffic Act and of the provisions that apply to A & E Departments.

When the driver of a motor vehicle is brought to hospital for examination and treatment after an accident, the Police Officer in charge of the case will request permission to carry out a breathalyser test on the patient. This test is for screening and, if it indicates that the blood alcohol may be too high, the patient will then be required to provide a blood specimen on which an accurate measurement of the alcohol level can be made. This may, if the level is below 80 mg per cent, help the patient; unfortunately, in many cases the level is well over 80 mg per cent and, when used in the subsequent legal proceedings, results in a conviction.

The Police Officer should always request permission from the doctor before approaching the patient to carry out a breathalyser test. The doctor must give permission if the patient's condition would not be adversely affected by the procedure. It should be refused if the patient is unconscious or suffering from injuries which would prevent the test being carried out. These include facial or chest injuries which would prevent the breathalyser bag being blown up during expiration. Severe shock, haemorrhage or major injuries would also be contra-indications but, provided the injuries are not major, it is not necessary that the patient should be uninjured.

If permission for the test is refused, the matter is closed. If it is considered that the patient is fit to undergo the test, the doctor should explain to the patient: 'This officer has asked me if he can carry out a breathalyser test on you. In my opinion you are fit to undergo the test and I have given him my permission to approach you for this purpose. He will explain the law to you, as I have no further involvement in the matter.'

Despite the apparent simplicity of the procedure, the doctor may still find himself in court giving evidence for the defence or prosection, and certain precautions are advisable to avoid this happening.

When the patient refuses the breathalyser and/or the provision of a blood sample, if the breathalyser is positive he may be charged with refusing to provide the specimen and may claim that, because of his injuries, he was not aware of what he was doing. The doctor must, therefore, satisfy himself that the patient is able to understand what was explained to him by the doctor and what was requested by the Police Officer. Clearly, an unconscious or badly confused patient with a head injury will have no understanding, but an inebriated patient may present difficulties from the cognitive aspect. It is advisable that the doctor records his decision about permission or refusal for the test and the reasons for this decision on the case sheet. In this way, if questions of the patient's fitness are raised at a later date by either side, the doctor is in a position to give a reasoned answer to the questions and may avoid the necessity to give evidence in court.

If the breathalyser test is positive, the police will contact a police surgeon and ask him to come to the hospital to take a blood sample. Permission for this may be refused on medical grounds but, if the initial permission for the breathalyser was correct, there should be no reason why a blood test cannot be carried out. The police surgeon will bring his own equipment for the blood test. The hospital, apart from providing the space in which the test may be carried out, must take no part in the proceedings. They must not help or make any equipment or material of any nature available for the test. If equipment has been forgotten, it should not be made available from the hospital. The law lays down that the hospital must take no part in the procedure and, if they do, any legal proceedings may fail because of this unlawful assistance.

It is equally unlawful for persons to be brought specifically to the hospital solely for the purpose of taking a blood sample. Drivers who do not need to be brought to hospital on medical grounds must have all the procedures carried out at the scene of the incident and at the local police station. Any attempt to use the hospital for the purposes of the Road Traffic Act and not for the purpose of diagnosis and treatment must be refused. In these cases the doctor must be careful not to appear to associate himself with either the patient or the Police Officer in the proceedings required by the Road Traffic Act. He has 3 decisions to make:

1. Is the patient fit or unfit to be interviewed?
2. Is the patient fit to provide a specimen of breath?
3. Is the patient fit to provide a specimen of blood or urine?

Once these decisions have been made, both the doctor and the hospital have no further part to play and the situation must be resolved between the patient and the Police Officer without outside assistance.

Appendix I

TELEPHONE NUMBERS OF POISONS INFORMATION CENTRES

Belfast	0232–40503
Cardiff	0222–33101
Dublin	Eire Dublin 45588
Edinburgh	031–229–2477
Leeds	0532–32799
London	01–407–7600
Manchester	061–740–2254

Appendix II

Potassium dihydrogen orthophosphate   350 g
Disodium hydrogen orthophosphate (hydrated 12.H_2O)   900 g
Sterile water to 5 litres
Pack in 500 ml MRC bottles and sterilize by autoclaving.

This solution can be used for topical irrigation of the eyes and mouth.
It should be used only with strongly ionizing caustic and alkaline radicals.
It is **not** intended for intravenous use.

The solution may be obtained from Macarthys Pharmaceuticals, Romford, Essex.

Appendix III

DESFERRIOXAMINE DROPS FOR RUST RINGS IN THE EYE

These should be freshly made up for each patient and have a shelf-life of 7 days when stored under refrigeration.
Two to three drops should be applied every 2 or 3 hours.
These drops should be prepared in the pharmacy using injection of Desferal and Hypromellose eye drops, the formulation being 5 ml of Hypromellose drops to 500 mg of Desferal injection, using an aseptic technique.

Appendix IV

BIBLIOGRAPHY FOR POISON REFERENCES

The following books are suitable as reference sources for the treatment of poisoning:

Poisoning by Drugs and Chemicals, Cooper, P., published by Alchemist, 1974

Treatment of Common Acute Poisonings, Matthew and Lawson, published by Churchill Livingstone, 1975

Martindale, The Extra Pharmacopoeia, edited by Wade, A., published by the Pharmaceutical Press, 27th edition, 1977

Clinical Toxicology of Commercial Products, Gleason, M. N., Gosselin, R. E., Hodge, H. C. and Smith, R. P., published by the Williams and Wilkins Company, Baltimore, 1969

Clinical Toxicology, Polson, C. J. and Tattersall, R. N., published by Pitman Medical Publishing Company Limited, 1969

Psychotropic Drugs: A Manual for Emergency Management of Overdose, Kilne, N. S., Alexander, S. F. and Chamberlain, A., published by the Medical Economics Company, Oradell, New Jersey, 1974

Mushrooms and Toadstools in Colour, Else and Hands Hvass, published by Blandford Press, 1970

Poisonous Plants and Fungi, North, P., published by Blandford Press, 1967

ABPI (Associaition of the British Pharmaceutical Industry) Data Sheet Compendium, published annually by Pharmind

Mims. Monthly Index of Medical Specialities, published monthly by Haymarket Publishing Limited, London

British Poisonous Plants, Forsyth, A. A., Bulletin 161, published by HMSO, 1968

Dangerous Properties of Industrial Materials, Sax N.I. *et al.,* published by Van Nostrand Reinhold Company, New York and London, 1968

Drug Interactions, Hansten, P. D., published by Lea and Febiger, 1973

Approved Products for Farmers and Growers, Ministry of Agriculture, Fisheries and Food, published annually by HMSO

A Paediatric Vade Mecum, edited by Wood, B., published by Lloyd Luke (Medical Books) Limited, 1974

Transport Emergency Cards, published by the Chemical Industries Association Limited

Carriage of Dangerous Substances by Road, Department of Health and Social Security Health Notice, HN(77)167. This circular, together with the new schedule, covers a very large number of hazardous products and gives appropriate advice, where necessary, on the uses and hazards of the substances. Protective measures are indicated where appropriate.

Index